From Supraventricular Tachycardias to Cardiac Resynchronization Therapy

Edited by Gabriel Cismaru

Published in London, United Kingdom

From Supraventricular Tachycardias to Cardiac Resynchronization Therapy
http://dx.doi.org/10.5772/intechopen.111303
Edited by Gabriel Cismaru

Contributors
Abdullah Dhawi Al-Otaibi, Abdulmohsen Almusaad, Abdulrahman Abdullatif Alarfaj, Adil Baimbetov, Ahmed Bander Alsalem, Ahmed Hussein, Cynthia M. Tracy, Dorys Chavez, Faisal Rabeea Alananzi, Jamal A. Masri, Luis Cerna Urrutia, Malik Ghawanmeh, Mareyah Alshaikh Husain, Muneera AlTaweel, Rabya S. Saraf, Radu Darciuc, Rafael J. Ramirez, Rasmah Saad Alharajin, Samuel J. Bergman, Sarah AlMukhaylid, Somshukla Ghosh, Yousef Alanazi, Zainab Albahrani

First published in London, United Kingdom, 2024 by IntechOpen
IntechOpen is the global imprint of INTECHOPEN LIMITED, registered in England and Wales, registration number: 11086078, 167-169 Great Portland Street, London, W1W 5PF, United Kingdom

British Library Cataloguing-in-Publication Data
A catalogue record for this book is available from the British Library

Additional hard and PDF copies can be obtained from orders@intechopen.com

From Supraventricular Tachycardias to Cardiac Resynchronization Therapy
Edited by Gabriel Cismaru
p. cm.

This title is part of the Cardiology and Cardiovascular Medicine Book Series, Volume 5
Topic: Cardiovascular Electrophysiology
Series Editor: Kaan Kırali
Topic Editor: Karine Guerrier

Print ISBN 978-0-85466-788-8
Online ISBN 978-0-85466-787-1
eBook (PDF) ISBN 978-0-85466-789-5
ISSN 3033-361X

For EU product safety concerns:
IN TECH d.o.o., Prolaz Marije Krucifikse Kozulić 3, 51000 Rijeka, Croatia, info@intechopen.com or visit our website at intechopen.com.

IntechOpen Book Series

Cardiology and Cardiovascular Medicine

Volume 5

Aims and Scope of the Series

Today, since molecular science on structural causes of oncological pathologies and their molecular treatments are developing at an unbelievable rate, the primary medical cause of death in the twenty-first century will be cardiovascular disease. Neither pandemics that threaten all humanity nor deterioration in the ecosystem will be able to change this fact. Especially, this century seems poised to witness an incredible struggle against atherosclerotic disease, which develops in the arterial walls and results in narrowing and occlusion of the arterial lumen. In addition to this disease, there has been an increasing prevalence of heart rhythm problems, deterioration of heart valves due to aging, and heart failure. Serious vascular pathologies such as stenosis and occlusion, dissection and rupture, and aneurysmal enlargement are also major concerns. Medical and invasive treatment methods may work to save human lives, but they will never provide a real solution. All kinds of medical, technological, and genetic engineering developments obtained in these processes have not yet been sufficient to alleviate or eliminate cardiovascular disease. This book series, Cardiology and Cardiovascular Medicine, includes three topics. The first, Cardiovascular Diseases and Health, reviews important cardiovascular diseases and the developments in their prognosis. The second topic, Cardiovascular Electrophysiology, illuminates the abnormal functioning of the cardiac conduction system, which is caused by all heart pathologies and negatively affects prognosis. The third topic in this series, Cardiovascular Surgery, details treatment for cardiovascular pathologies and how to regulate normal physiological functions with percutaneous or extracorporeal interventions.

Meet the Series Editor

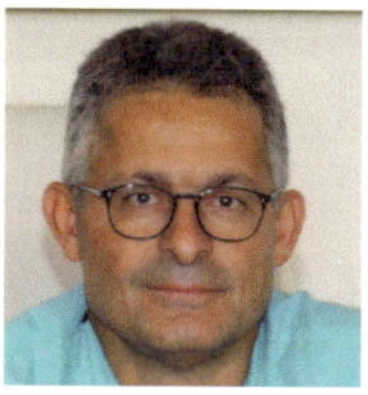

After completing his studies at the Medicine Faculty of Istanbul University in 1990, Prof. Kaan Kırali fulfilled his mandatory medical service and commenced his residency training at Koşuyolu Heart and Research Hospital in 1992. Following five years of assistant education, he pursued further training in England and the USA in 1998. Specializing in laparoscopic and minimally invasive cardiac surgery, he earned the titles of consultant cardiovascular surgeon in 1998, Assistant Professor in 1999, Associate Professor in 2002, and Chief in 2005 at the same hospital. Prof. Kırali also developed an interest in preventive medicine, obtaining an MSc in Public Health from Istanbul University in 2000. Over the past two decades, he has concentrated his scientific pursuits on cardiovascular repairs requiring specialized experience. With his expertise in coronary artery surgery, minimally invasive cardiac surgery, valve repair, and aortic root surgery, he has established new methods for awake coronary bypass revascularization, a new surgical approach for AVR during first and re-operations, aortic valve-sparing procedure, and radiofrequency ablation. Notably, he pioneered awake complete coronary artery bypass grafting (CABG) with bilateral internal mammary arteries (BIMA) and played a crucial role in advancing aortic root surgery with a new aortotomy incision, simplifying aortic valve interventions. Since the year 2000, Prof. Kırali has expanded his interests to heart transplantation, and in recent years, to left ventricular assist devices. He has served as the head of the transplantation department since 2015 and currently continues his work as the director of Koşuyolu High Specialization Education and Research Hospital in Istanbul, Turkey. In his prolific career, he has authored numerous papers in SCI journals, contributed to various book chapters, and served as an editor and reviewer for multiple academic journals. Additionally, he has edited several international books in the field of cardiovascular medicine.

Meet the Volume Editor

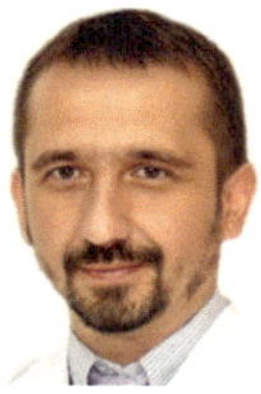

Dr. Cismaru completed his medical degree in 2005 at UMF Cluj-Napoca, Romania, and currently practices in the Electrophysiology Laboratory at the Rehabilitation Hospital in Cluj. After achieving specialization in the field of cardiology, he successfully finished his fellowship in cardiac electrophysiology at the Institut Lorrain du Coeur et des Vaisseaux Louis Mathieu in CHU de Nancy, France. While in France, he developed expertise in doing catheter ablation procedures for atrial fibrillation and ventricular tachycardia. After obtaining the European certification in cardiac electrophysiology from the European Heart Rhythm Association (EHRA) in 2015, he broadened his practice to the implantation of cardiac devices such as pacemakers, internal defibrillators, loop recorders, and resynchronization devices. In 2016, he achieved EHRA certification in cardiac pacing. His main focus is on cardiac arrhythmias in both adults and children.

Contents

Preface

This book addresses two distinct clinical situations: patients with supraventricular arrhythmias and patients with dyssynchrony who would benefit from resynchronization therapy for improving heart failure treatment. Evidently, these two subjects exhibit disparities; however, they share certain fundamental components. Hence, the connection between supraventricular arrhythmias and resynchronization therapy is not coincidental. On one hand, certain persistent atrial arrhythmias can cause the left ventricle to enlarge, a condition known as tachyarrhythmic cardiomyopathy. On the other hand, dilated cardiomyopathy can be further complicated by arrhythmias, particularly supraventricular ones like atrial fibrillation. Prior to initiating any resynchronization therapy, it is necessary to address the atrial arrhythmia in order to ensure a high pacing percentage and establish optimal cardiac synchronization.

The first section of the book focuses on supraventricular arrhythmias: from tachycardias caused by accessory pathways to atrial fibrillation.

The second section of the book addresses the physiological justification and technique of resynchronization therapy in patients with heart failure, as well as indications, implantation techniques, complications, and long-term outcomes.

In the first chapter Adil Baimbetov describes accessory pathways and the types of reentrant arrhythmias that can be induced in this category of patients. Orthodromic atrioventricular reentrant tachycardia (AVRT) frequently develops in the presence of an accessory pathway (AP) that conducts retrogradely. The pathogenic impulse travels from atria to ventricles through the normal atrioventricular conduction system, while it travels backward to the atria using the retrograde conducting accessory pathway. Occasionally, conduction takes place in the opposite direction, leading to the occurrence of antidromic AVRT with a large QRS complex. Accessory pathways can be found at any location along the atrioventricular rings, either mitral or tricuspid, and are typically solitary abnormalities. However, in certain individuals, congenital defects such as Ebstein anomaly or transposition of great arteries may also be present. The majority of accessory pathways exhibit nondecremental conduction characteristics and are conducted at a faster rate compared to normal atrioventricular conduction tissue. This gives a risk of ventricular fibrillation in case of atrial fibrillation conducted anterogradely to the ventricle. Baseline electrocardiogram in a significant number of individuals with accessory pathways shows preexcitation, recognized by a short PR interval and a delta wave at the beginning of the QRS. Special algorithms can be used to predict the location of the pathways. Electrophysiological studies are frequently conducted in these patients with the aim of diagnosis, localization, and identification of the risk of sudden death related to the accessory pathway. In recent decades, catheter ablation has arisen as a radical therapy option for patients with Wolf–Parkinson–White (WPW) syndrome. The authors describe different techniques for catheter ablation using either radiofrequency or criotherapy, guided by X-ray or three-dimensional mapping techniques. This presentation, prepared by the authors, is highly helpful as it thoroughly explores the intricate details of the accessory pathways, encompassing every detail from the mechanism to the therapy.

In the second chapter, Rafael J. Ramirez et al. provide a comprehensive assessment of animal and computer models used to study atrial fibrillation (AF)—models that have generated useful insights into the mechanism of this arrhythmia. These models play a crucial role in bridging the gap between nonclinical and clinical research and have proved vital in improving our understanding of the various factors that contribute to the progression of cardiac arrhythmia. Researchers employ several investigative methods and scientific models to obtain understanding of the factors that influence the initiation and advancement of atrial fibrillation. They also evaluate new treatments and therapeutic techniques through experimentation. Both large and small animal models, along with computational techniques, are extremely helpful tools for enhancing our understanding of this arrhythmia. Animal models give a biological background and empirical evidence, while computational models offer a versatile platform for evaluating theories and analyzing data. The combined use of these two methodologies enables a more thorough comprehension of AF. The integration of experimental and theoretical approaches will be increasingly vital in the development of effective drugs and the attainment of a comprehensive understanding of atrial fibrillation, as technology and materials continue to advance.

Cardiac resynchronization therapy (CRT) has emerged as a crucial treatment for individuals suffering from severe heart failure and left bundle branch block in recent decades. The presence of a large QRS complex is a sign of dyssynchrony between the left ventricle and the right ventricle, causing a reduction in the ejection fraction. Correcting the dyssynchrony by synchronizing the two ventricles is an effective therapy for increasing the left ventricular ejection fraction.

Abdulmohsen Almusaad et al. provide a concise overview of the development, performance, scientific studies, criteria for selecting patients, handling, and improvement of cardiac resynchronization therapy. The main topics discussed include recommendations for the use of CRT, both invasive and noninvasive imaging methods to improve results, various pacing locations to optimize response, and advancements in lead technology and implantation techniques. The chapter emphasizes the areas where our understanding is lacking and suggests future research topics to enhance the use of CRT and clinical results in real-world settings. By conducting additional research to address any remaining uncertainties, it is quite likely that CRT will become an even more efficient treatment for heart failure patients with dyssynchronous cardiomyopathy. The progression of cardiac resynchronization therapy CRT from its early experimental phases to a widely accepted treatment for heart failure with reduced ejection fraction and ventricular dyssynchrony has been amazing. Cardiac resynchronization therapy CRT has unquestionably transformed the field of heart failure treatment, resulting in a reduction of symptoms, an improvement in quality of life, and an enhancement in survival rates. The efficacy of cardiac resynchronization therapy CRT in reversing negative remodeling and improving heart function has been demonstrated in trials and other significant investigations.

Malik Ghawanmeh et al. analyze the recommendations on CRT in individuals with heart failure. In their chapter, they investigate the current understanding of CRT responders by examining the most recent evidence. They investigate the influence of

CRT on mortality rates, hospitalizations due to heart failure, clinical characteristics of heart failure, preservation of ventricular function, and preventing the advancement of heart failure. They explore the most recent progress in physiological pacing, which includes studying the anatomical and physiological characteristics, while carefully assessing the benefits and disadvantages. In addition, the chapter examines potential future opportunities and directions in this field, offering a comprehensive picture of the developing potential of CRT. Extensive study over many years has resulted in significant advancements in understanding the relationship between cardiac conduction anomalies, symptoms, morbidity, and mortality. Significant progress has been achieved in correcting electromechanical dyssynchrony. The data strongly supports the benefits of CRT in specific patients with symptomatic heart failure with reduced ejection fraction and electrical dyssynchrony. Cardiac resynchronization therapy improves quality of life and decreases mortality. When CRT is not practical, conduction system pacing offers a viable alternative. Attractive options lie in future developments of the technique, patient selection, and companies' innovations.

Radu Darciuc provides a comprehensive overview of the key technical considerations required for the implantation of CRT devices. It includes many procedures such as anesthesia, venous access, creation of the pocket, cannulation of the coronary sinus, and implantation of the left ventricular lead. A description of the necessary equipment is provided to assist implanting physicians in getting familiar with and overcoming potential problems throughout the procedure. Darciuc evaluates multiple techniques for every stage, highlighting their strengths and weaknesses. He provides an extensive set of tips and techniques that will assist physicians in conducting implantations with greater skill and expertise. The description of the technique is enhanced by the inclusion of numerous figures and images, which provide a more comprehensive understanding of the procedure. Implanting a CRT device is a complex technique that involves multiple successive steps. In the absence of adequate preparation and training, there may arise huge challenges that are hard to surmount. Electrophysiology specialists should develop plans of action for each individual challenge encountered during cardiac resynchronization therapy setup. Developing an effective strategy is crucial for successfully addressing all obstacles.

Finally, but not least, Somshukla Ghosh et al. examine clinical trials that focused on the impact of several treatments on reducing mortality in patients with cardiomyopathy and heart failure. The treatments investigated were CRT with a pacemaker (CRT-P), internal cardiac defibrillator (ICD) alone, and a combination of CRT and ICD (CRT-D). A CRT device, specifically a CRT-P device without a defibrillator, has the potential to effectively decrease mortality rates in these individuals. On the other hand, defibrillators that do not include CRT have been employed to decrease mortality in the same group of patients. For patients with left bundle branch block, cardiomyopathy, and a reduced ejection fraction (LVEF) of 35 percent or less, it is recommended to consider using a cardiac resynchronization therapy with defibrillator (CRT-D) device, as long as there are no reasons to avoid defibrillation therapy. This treatment option may offer the greatest reduction in mortality, potentially due to a decreased risk of death from arrhythmias when using this combination. However, CRT-P has demonstrated advantages that extend beyond just alleviating heart failure symptoms and enhancing quality of life. It also offers a substantial reduction in mortality, making it a viable option when defibrillation therapy is not recommended.

Overall, these chapters provide valuable information for experienced cardiologists specializing in arrhythmology, both electrophysiologists and device implantation doctors. They cover the treatment of supraventricular arrhythmias through ablation, as well as the challenging technique of CRT implantation. This book is intended to be beneficial to you all.

Gabriel Cismaru
Cardiology Department,
Iuliu Hatieganu University of Medicine and Pharmacy,
Cluj-Napoca, Romania

Section 1

Supraventricular Tachycardias

Chapter 1

Tachycardias Associated with Accessory Pathways: Mechanisms and Catheter Ablation

Adil Baimbetov

Abstract

Accessory pathways (AP) of abnormal conduction are pathways between the ventricular and atrial myocardium that exist apart from the conduction system structures. Patients with AP of abnormal atrioventricular conduction may have ventricular tachycardia known as atrioventricular (AV) reciprocating tachycardia (AVRT). Orthodromic AVRT often occurs in the presence of AP. The pathological impulse passes antegrade via the normal AV conduction system, whereas retrograde conduction to the atria via AP. Rarely, conduction occurs in the opposite direction, resulting in antidromic AVRT. APs occur at all points of the AV ring and usually as isolated anomalies, although in some patients, congenital anomalies are observed. Most APs have non-decremental conduction properties and are conducted more rapidly than normal tissue with AV conduction. In many patients with AP, baseline ECG reveals clear preexcitation signs and special algorithms can be used to presume their localization. Electrophysiologic study in these patients is often performed with in the purpose of diagnosing, localizing, and determining AP's functional characteristics. Drug therapy for AVRT prevention is useful for temporary control while waiting for drastic actions and, in some cases, for long-term treatment. Over the last few decades, a radical treatment option as catheter ablation has emerged in patient's treatment with WPW syndrome.

Keywords: accessory pathway, catheter treatment, radiofrequency ablation, accessory pathway ablation, concealed pathway

1. Introduction

Accessory pathways are tracts formed by modified myocardiocytes or cells of the cardiac conduction system, connecting the myocardium of the atria and ventricles or various parts of the cardiac conduction system. Being morphologically similar to the tracts of the conduction system, APs have higher conductivity. As a result of their functioning, pre-excitation of the ventricles is formed, and tachyarrhythmias occur, which often have hemodynamic significance. APs are the morphological substrate of Wolff–Parkinson–White (WPW) syndrome. WPW syndrome is the most common congenital heart disease, and supraventricular tachycardias (SVT) that occur with this syndrome are rarely associated with life-threatening conditions. Still, despite this, they are the most common reason for seeking emergency medical care. Drug therapy for this pathology cannot radically help such patients; resistance to antiarrhythmic drugs develops in 56–70% of patients within 1–5 years. Timely diagnosis and treatment of AVRT in WPW syndrome is an urgent problem in clinical cardiology since it develops at working age in most cases. The radiofrequency ablation (RFA) of the APs has become widespread due to its safety and high efficiency in treating patients with AVRT. Today, it is generally accepted that radiofrequency catheter ablation of the additional atrioventricular junction is a highly effective method of treating WPW syndrome, characterized by a low risk of complications and thereby ensuring the return of patients to normal, full-fledged life activities.

2. Accessory pathways of cardiac conduction system

F. Wood et al. first described accessory pathways (APs) of the cardiac conduction system during histologic examination of a deceased patient's heart with WPW syndrome. Shortly after, its most accurate description was given by R. Ohnell, who found that the accessory pathways are "thin threads" of atrial myocardium. According to the data obtained by A. Becker et al. in 1978, the APs are thicker at their origin in the atrium. Spreading in the ventricular myocardium, they branch like tree roots [1–3]. Histologically, they are fibers, typically consisting of working atrial myocardium, located at various depths in the fatty tissue of the atrial-ventricular sulcus and connect the atrial and ventricular myocardium. The thickness of these bundles ranges from 0.1 to 7 mm (1.3 mm on average). In accordance with the anatomical classification of APs, "connection" refers to abnormal conductive pathways penetrating the contractile ventricular myocardium, and "tract" refers to abnormal pathways terminating in specialized conductive tissue [4–6].

The main ones are the following:

1. Atrioventricular (AV) pathways ("Kent bundles").

2. Nodoventricular tract between the AV pathway and the right side of the interventricular septum (Mahaim fibers).

3. Nodofascicular tract between AV pathway and the branching of the right branch of the His bundle (Mahaim fibers).

4. Fasciculoventricular junction between the common His bundle and the myocardium of the right ventricle (Mahaim fibers). Generally, it functions in rare cases.

5. Atriofascicular tract connecting the right atrium to the common His bundle (Breschenmacher tract). It tends to be rare.

6. Atrionodal tract between the SA node and the inferior part of the AV pathway (posterior inter-nodal James tract). This tract is present in all humans but is usually non-functional (**Figure 1**).

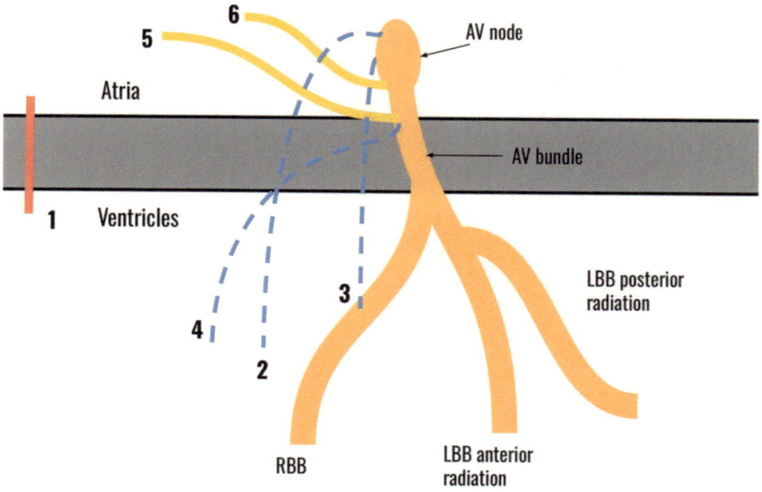

Figure 1.
The figure illustrates possible types of existing AP. A description is given in the text (above).

The Breschenmacher tract and the posterior inter-nodal James tract are also called the AV nodal bypasses since they allow sinus or atrial impulses to reach the common His bundle without delay at the AV junction. The same category includes so-called short pathways in the AV node, along with "small" and "underdeveloped" AV nodes. The above classification does not reflect concealed retrograde "Kent bundles" and multiple APs [7, 8]. Accessory atrioventricular pathways can be located at any point of the atrial-ventricular sulcus except for the area between the aorta and the mitral valve ring. They are commonly divided into parietal and septal. The first one attaches to the free walls of the left and right ventricles, and the others connect the interatrial septum with the interventricular septum, terminating anteriorly or posteriorly in its membranous part, in the right triangle of the central fibrous body, generally under the endocardium near the typical structures of the conduction system. W. Untereker et al. (1980) summarized the anatomical data available in the literature on the hearts of 35 deceased patients whose ECG registered signs of WPW syndrome during life. Short (1 to 10 mm) and narrow (average diameter - 1.3 mm) muscle bundles starting in the lower atrial regions and penetrating into the ventricular muscle were found in 30 cases. In most cases, left-sided APs were located outside the compact, well-formed fibrous mitral annulus and crossed the fatty layer of the epicardial sulcus close to it. Right-sided APs pass to the ventricular myocardium through congenital disabilities "gaps" of the tricuspid fibrous ring, whose backbone is "weaker". There are also superficial APs lying distant from the fibrous rings in the fatty tissue of the venous sulcus. In 1986, G. Guiraudon et al. showed that posterior-septal APs can connect the left ventricle's posterior part with the right atrium's adjacent part [9–11]. In 1988, W. Jackman, based on the analysis of delta wave morphology in 12 standard leads of the surface ECG and fluoroscopy localization, proposed to distinguish the following APs in WPW syndrome:

1. Septal APs: - right anterior or anterior-septal; – right medial-septal; – right posterior-septal; – left posterior-septal; – subepicardial.

2. Right APs: - right; – anterolateral; – lateral.

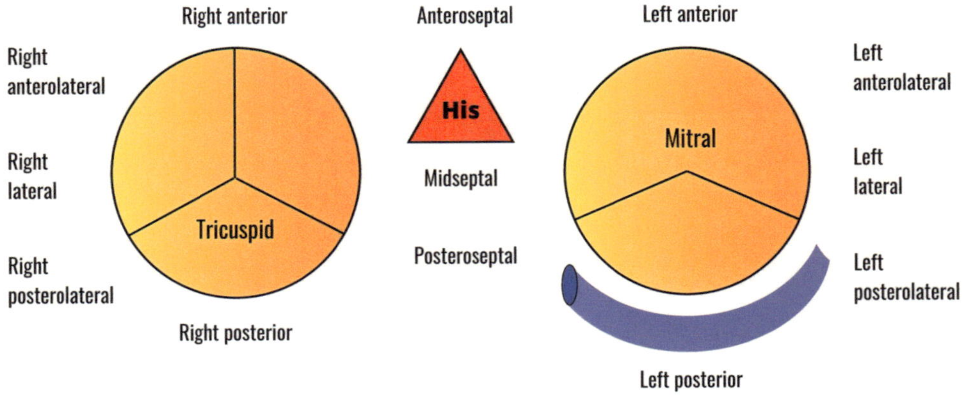

Figure 2.
Generally accepted classification of AP localization.

3. Left-sided APs: - anterolateral; – lateral; – posterior. Considering the anatomical location of the heart in the thorax, in 1999, F.G. Cosio proposed an anatomical classification of localization of accessory atrioventricular pathways in WPW syndrome. This classification divides all WPWs into right-sided, left-sided, and paraseptal (**Figure 2**)

Accessory pathways also can be divided in accordance with their location, direction, arrhythmia mechanism, and conduction characteristics.

Further, according to the anatomical properties they are subdivided into septal, left-sided, and right-sided conduction pathways. Posterior septal, medial septal, and anteroseptal can be combined into septal pathways, and left-/right-sided pathways can be subdivided into posterior, posterolateral, lateral, anterolateral, and anterior.

Several accessory pathways may be located in unusual anatomical spots, such as the epicardial connections between the left ventricle and the coronary sinus, the left ventricle and the noncoronary cusp of the aortic valve, the right ventricle and the right atrial appendage, or the left ventricle and the left atrial appendage. In addition, a few accessory pathways may be connected to a specialized conducting system straightaway, such as fasciculoventricular, nodofascicular, and atriofascicular pathways.

Accessory pathways also can be characterized in accordance with their conduction direction (e.g., retrograde, anterograde, or bidirectional - see above), or according to their conductive features. Regarding the latter, most accessory pathways have fast, non-decremental conduction, but some paraseptal pathways might have slow or decremental conduction, the same as the AV node.

3. Mechanisms of arrhythmias involving accessory pathways

The first classification of arrhythmia mechanisms was presented in 1964: (1) impulse formation disturbance, (2) impulse conduction disorders, and (3) their combinations. These works were based on studies on the transmembrane potential of cardiomyocytes.

As a rule, most myocardium and conduction system cells have negative resting potential (−80 mV). Exceptions are cells of the sinus node (SN), atrioventricular node (AVN), and atrioventricular valve area, where resting potential is higher

(−70 mV). A negative potential on the membrane surface is due to a potassium gradient associated with the potassium-sodium pump's function. The depolarization phase of the cell is due to the exit of sodium ions from the cell, and the "plateau" phase is due to the slow exit of calcium and potassium entry. Automatism or spontaneous generation of impulses is caused by phase 4 of depolarization, which can be suppressed by overdrive pacing, as the potassium-sodium pump, in this case, leads to the cell hyperpolarization [12, 13].

Impulse conduction disorders are caused by the presence of cells with pathological resting potential and slowly increasing action potential (induced by calcium ion current) or by disruption in intercellular contacts (desmosomes). These factors create conditions for conduction delay and macroreentry formation. The formation of an unidirectional blockade in a system of multiple myocardial fibres may also lead to the development of excitation re-entry or macroreentry. In 1983, the possibility of re-entry formation in a small area of the atrial border ridge was demonstrated, even in the presence of anisotropy [4, 12].

Excitation re-entry wave underlies most tachyarrhythmias. The rhythm of heartbeats arising from this conduction disturbance is caused by electric current circulation in the myocardial area, leading to periodic depolarization of the cardiomyocyte membrane.

Under normal conditions, impulses from the sinus node propagate through the myocardium in a strictly ordered manner, after which they decay. Each section of the conducting system and each region of the myocardium is depolarized under the action of a single excitation impulse only once (due to the refractoriness of cells preventing tissue reactivation immediately after the impulse passage) [13]. The mechanism of the excitation re-entry wave is shown in **Figure 3**.

This circle can exist indefinitely, with each impulse passage activating distal parts of the conducting system, after which the excitation wave propagates throughout the myocardium, causing tachyarrhythmias. Theoretically, retrograde conduction slowing is not a prerequisite for the existence of the re-entry mechanism. The excitation wave re-entry is possible only if the propagating impulse reaches cells whose membrane can be depolarized. Consequently, the pulse travel time through the re-entry circuit must be longer than the refractory period of the excitable tissue. If the re-entry circuit transit time is less than this period, the impulse will fade after reaching the refractory tissue [14]. As a rule, the pulse conduction velocity is about 50 cm/s, and the duration of the refractory period is −200 ms. Obviously, for the realization of the re-entry mechanism, the circuit length should be at least 10 cm. However, in practice, the circulation of excitation impulses is observed in much smaller areas

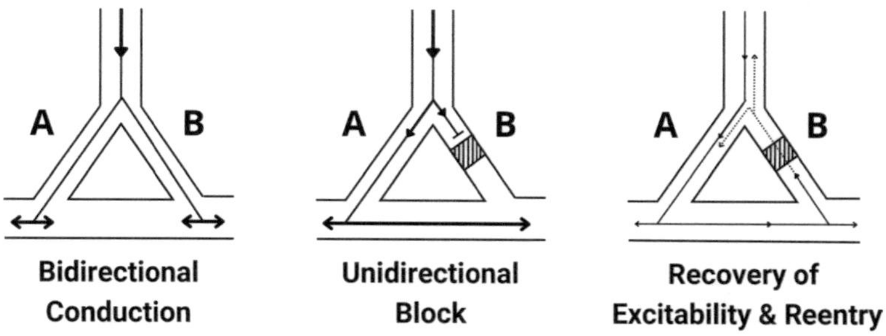

Figure 3.
The primary mechanism of arrhythmia with the participation of the AP is re-entry.

of the myocardium, so retrograde impulse conduction slowing down is still necessary in most cases to develop the re-entry mechanism and persistent heart rhythm disruption.

Thus, two conditions are necessary to develop a mechanism of the excitation wave re-entry: (1) unilateral conduction blockade and (2) slowing of impulse conduction along the re-entry circuit. Compliance with these conditions is possible if neighboring cells differ in the rate of impulse conduction and the refractory period duration [15].

A classic example of an arrhythmia re-entry is orthodromic or antidromic atrial-ventricular tachycardia involving an accessory conduction pathway. Due to its abnormal location, this bundle links the atrial myocardium to the ventricular myocardium (**Figure 4**). The accessory pathway conducts the impulse rapidly, and the typical delay of the excitation wave in the AV node does not occur. Consequently, the ventricles are excited earlier than usual, accompanied by a shortening of the P-R interval on the ECG (usually less than 0.12 sec). Moreover, in such individuals, ventricular depolarization is caused by impulses from both the AV node and the accessory conduction pathway. As a result, vast QRS complexes with earlier than regular rise in the initial complex part are observed on ECG. There are many variations in the severity of the delta wave (ventricular preexcitation) (depending on the electrophysiologic properties of WPW and AV node), up to its complete absence in patients with intermittent, latent, or latent WPW syndrome. Also, in these patients, there are signs of repolarization disruption in the form of various changes in the T waveform (due to atopic ventricular depolarization, the repolarization process is also atopic), which is often mistakenly interpreted as an ischemia manifestation [16].

The accessory conduction pathway is the anatomical basis of the long re-ventricular chain. The components of this circuit are, on the one hand, the accessory pathway and, on the other hand, the AV node. The conduction velocity and refractory period duration of the accessory and regular pathways usually differ, so appropriate frequency impulses can lead to tachyarrhythmias by the re-entry mechanism.

Under regular sinus rhythm, conduction can be antegrade down the AP or via the AV node, resulting in an obvious preexcitation on the ECG. Frequently, this might not be obvious in the case of the ventricle depolarization via the AV node before conduction via the accessory pathway is complete, as in a slow-conducting left lateral accessory pathway. This phenomenon is known as latent preexcitation because the 12-lead ECG during typical sinus rhythm might appear normal. In case accessory pathways

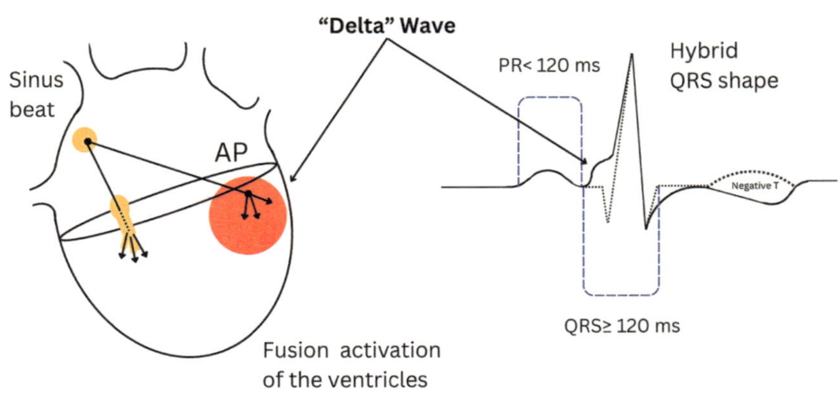

Figure 4.
Scheme of premature impulse conduction through the AP and the ventricle's preexcitation.

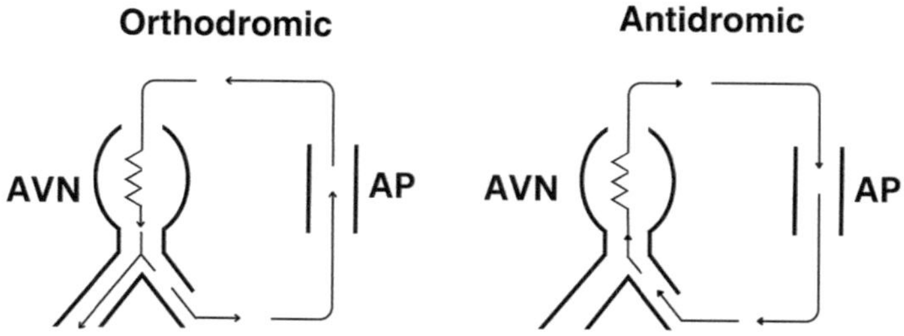

Figure 5.
Schemes of the orthodromic and antidromic tachycardia development with the AP participation. AVN- AV node, AP-accessory pathway.

conduct uniquely retrogradely during regular sinus rhythm, the ECG will also appear normal, and this is so-called concealed accessory conduction pathway. Concealed accessory conduction pathways are commonly regarded as less dangerous in terms of sudden death risk because they cannot conduct fast AF. Most accessory pathways have antegrade and retrograde properties [17].

If the antegrade accessory pathway is refractory and conduction takes place *antegradely* (via the AV node, which leads to the activation of His and the ventricle), and *retrogradely* (via the accessory pathway) Orthodromic AVRT takes place, which is illustrated in **Figure 5**. Typically, this occurs when the required VA time is greater than 70 ms. In spite of, insignificant changes in antegrade conduction via the AV node, the VA time, which indicates the time required for conduction via the accessory pathway, is usually steady and unchanged. In antidromic AVRT, conduction happens once the AV node is refractory, which favours antegrade conduction via the accessory pathway and retrograde atrial activation via the AV node and His, which is usually interconnected with QRS preexcitation because ventricular activation occurs only via the accessory pathway. Whereas conduction occurs via the AV node, the HA conduction time is typically more than 70 ms. This is more frequent in left lateral accessory pathways, as longer conduction times are required for the AV node to recover.

4. Electrophysiologic study of supraventricular tachycardias associated with accessory pathway of cardiac conduction system

Objectives of electrophysiologic study (EPS) in patients with supraventricular tachycardia (SVT) associated with accessory pathway of cardiac conduction system:

- verification of SVT-AVRT;
- management of its induction and determination modes;
- differential diagnosis with AVNRT, atrial and intra-atrial tachycardia, atrial fibrillation, and atrial flutter. In cases with antidromic tachycardia or AVRT with aberrant conduction along the His bundle branches, the differential diagnosis is carried out with ventricular tachycardia as well;
- obtaining information on the AP electrophysiological properties and determining its localization;

- determination of further treatment tactics;
- endocardial mapping of AP and RFCA.

Indications for EPS in patients with WPW syndrome are described in detail in the recommendations as 2019 ESC Guidelines for the management of patients with supraventricular tachycardia [18].

The study is performed in the X-ray operating room after withdrawal of all antiarrhythmic drugs for at least 6 half-lives.

Under local anesthesia, the left subclavian vein, right common femoral vein, and right femoral artery are punctured according to the Seldinger technique (in the case of left-sided localization of AP). 6–7 Fr diameter 2–3 introducers are inserted into the right common femoral vein. A 6 Fr diameter introducer is placed in the left subclavian vein and a 7 Fr in the right femoral artery (in left-sided localization of atrioventricular appendages).

Under X-ray control, diagnostic electrodes are placed in the coronary sinus (CS), His bundle region (HIS), and right ventricular apex (RVA) (**Figure 6**).

The protocol for EPS in patients with WPW syndrome includes evaluation of sinus node function recovery time, corrected sinus node function recovery time, anterograde and retrograde values of AP ERP and AV node, Wenckebach points, and verification of clinical AVRT (**Figure 7**). As a rule, APs are characterized by a nondecremental conduction.

The study includes the determination of the induction mode and clinical AVRT management (**Figure 8**). Frequently, in patients with WPW syndrome the VA interval exceeds 120 ms on the AVRT background. On intracardiac electrograms, the geometry of atrial myocardium retrograde activation will depend on the site of AP entry into the atrial myocardium. If the pulse propagates retrogradely along the left lateral AP, the earliest atrial activation will be observed in the distal regions of the CS from the

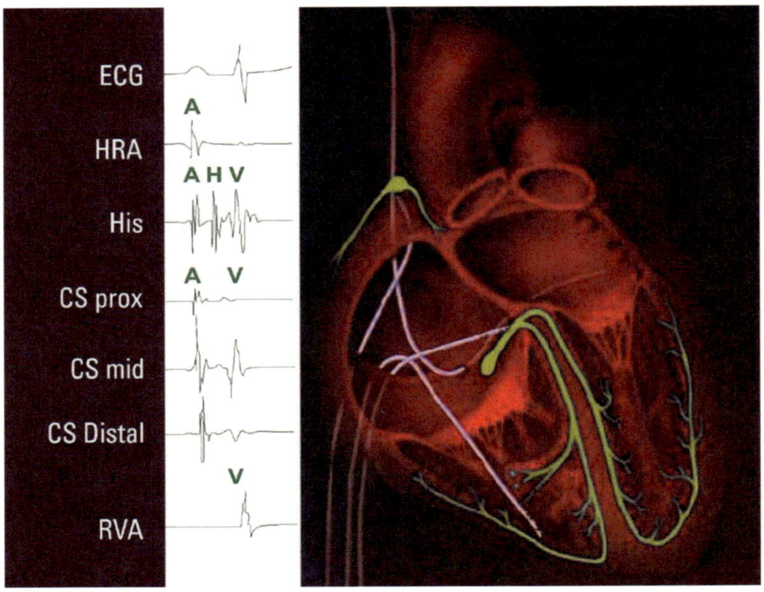

Figure 6.
Diagnostic electrode location during EP study and catheter ablation procedures, and recording electrograms.

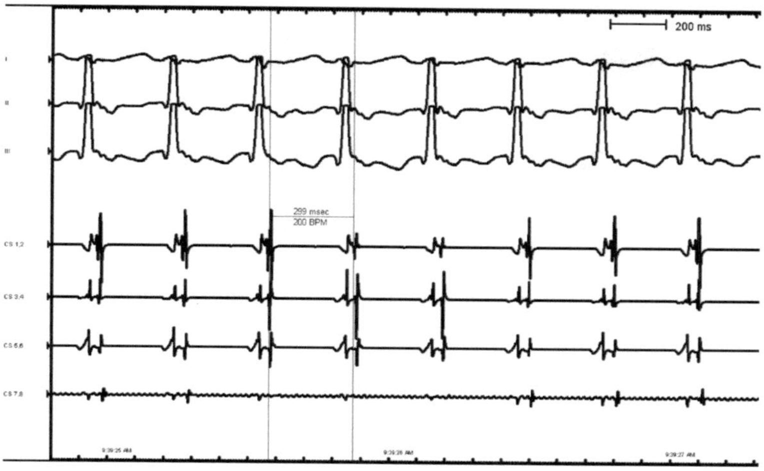

Figure 7.
Orthodromic tachycardia induction involving the AP left lateral localization during EP study.

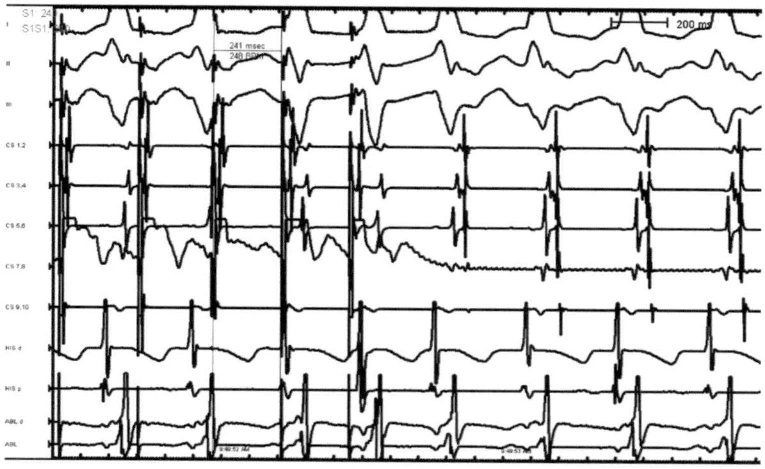

Figure 8.
Tachycardia induction with frequent pacing during EP study.

electrode pairs of the catheter located in the coronary sinus, in this case, CS1-2 (see **Figure 9**). On the orthodromic AVRT background in cases of functioning posterior or mid-septal APs, there is a "central type" of retrograde atrial activation, which complicates the differential diagnosis with atypical forms of AVNRT. In this case, to exclude AVNRT during the tachycardia paroxysm, the synchronized technique within 50 ms with the His bundle, ahead of the release of ventricular extrastimulus from the right ventricle apex is used. In typical or atypical AVNRT, synchronized extrastimulus (S2) does not alter the retrograde atrial activation geometry. The intervals during tachycardia (A-A, H-H) and after extrastimulus administration (A-ASt, H-HSt) remain identical because the extrastimulus cannot capture the atria as a result of the His bundle activation by the anterograde front and retrograde conduction is not possible. The H-H interval during tachycardia and after extrastimulus does not change,

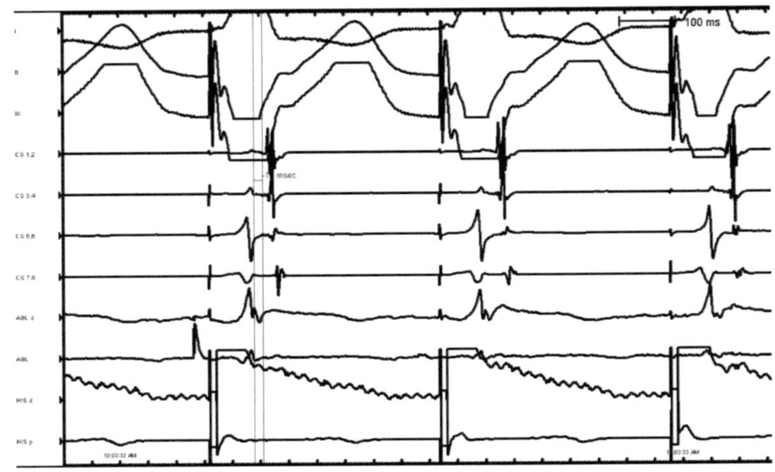

Figure 9.
The early point of atrial activation during retrograde pacing indicates the left anterior location of the AP.

indicating the absence of extrastimulus conduction through the His-Purkinje system. In case of retrograde conduction along the AP during a tachycardia paroxysm, the ventricular extrastimulus synchronized with the His bundle activation captures the atria. In this case, the electrogram reveals advancement of retrograde atrial activation (change of A-ASt intervals during tachycardia and after the administered extrastimulus). The earliest atrial activation is seen at the atrial output site of the AP. Premature ventricular extrastimulus can interrupt the paroxysm of AVRT. If there are difficulties in the differential diagnosis between AVNRT and AVRT, we recommend para-Hisian pacing to exclude concealed septal APs. The para-Hisian pacing stimulation technique is conducted in asynchronous pacing of ventricles with a cycle length of 500–600 ms from an area anatomically located close to the His bundle area (para-Hisian area). The electrophysiological properties of ventricular myocardium in this region differ significantly from those of the His bundle itself. At high values of current strength in the para-Hisian area, simultaneous capture of the His bundle or the proximal part of the His bundle right branch and adjacent contractile myocardium of the right ventricle occurs. On the baseline ECG, this is manifested by relatively narrow stimulation QRS complexes. Once the current is reduced or the patient breathes on the stimulating electrode, there might be a loss of the His bundle or right bundle branch capture, however, the capture of the contractile myocardium of the right ventricle is preserved (wide ventricular stimulation complexes are recorded on the ECG). In this case, the ventricular conduction system is activated retrogradely: first the ventricular myocardium and only then the Purkinje fibres - the His bundle legs - the His bundle. If the series of retrograde atrial activation does not change and the time intervals reflecting retrograde atrial activation remain unchanged in the case of trapping and non-trapping His-Purkinje complexes, then retrograde conduction via the concealed septal AP is assumed.

If there is no AP, retrograde conduction to the atria will depend on the direction of direct involvement of the His-Purkinje system elements in the retrograde activation circuit. In addition to the widening of the QRS complex, the absence of the His bundle "capture" will be accompanied by a prolongation of the interval illustrating retrograde activation of the atria. Thus, analysis of the retrograde atrial activation features on the para-Hisian stimulation in patients with SVT, first of all, allows differential diagnosis between atypical forms of AVNRT and orthodromic AVRT with the participation of retrogradely functioning septal APs. Occasionally, AV block of the second degree of Mobitz II may appear on the SVT background, which excludes AVRT as a cause of tachycardia. This phenomenon indicates that the maintenance of tachycardia does not require the involvement of underlying structures of the conducting system not involved in the loop of re-entry, such as the His bundle, the His bundle branch, and ventricular myocardium. In some cases, tachy-dependent blockade of impulse conduction along the His bundle branch is noted during an AVRT attack. As a rule, in this case, blockade of the His bundle branch on the side of the bundle location (ipsilateral blockade) prolongs the tachycardia cycle length and correspondingly decreases the ventricular activation rate, whereas in AVNRT the value of tachycardia cycle length before and after the onset of blockade does not change [19]. The differential diagnosis of AVNRT with "wide" QRS complexes during endocardial EPS is carried out primarily with ventricular tachycardias. Registration of endocardial electrograms from atria and ventricles greatly facilitates verification of ventricular-atrial dissociation during tachycardia based on different values of V-V and A-A intervals and makes the diagnosis of VT undoubted.

Differential diagnosis is also performed with SVT with wide QRS complexes. As a rule, this is not difficult in patients with antidromic AVRT and signs of preexcitation on the sinus rhythm (delta wave) background. During tachycardia the degree of their severity increases, because in this case, anterograde excitation of ventricles occurs only by AP, and retrograde - by the His-Purkinje system. In this case, the direction of the initial vector of ventricular depolarization in 12 leads of ECG will be the same both on the sinus rhythm background and during tachycardia. Difficulties may arise in the differential diagnosis of antidromic AVRT in a patient with no evidence of delta waves during sinus rhythm, which is sometimes observed in antidromic AVRT with anterograde conduction along the nodofascicular and nodoventricular tracts (Mahaim fibres). In such cases retrograde conduction is carried out by His-Purkinje system and analysis of atrial activation geometry will not clarify the situation completely. The sign characteristic for antidromic AVRT with anterograde conduction by Mahaim fibres is the change in the degree of pre-excitation depending on the cycle length of atrial pacing (the greater the frequency of atrial stimulation, the more pronounced the degree of ventricular pre-excitation) [20].

As a rule, the differential diagnosis of AVRT and atrial tachycardia is not difficult. The signs characterizing more atrial tachycardia than AVRT include the increase of PR interval during tachycardia, occurring at the shortening of tachycardia cycle length, appearance of AV blockade due to AAT administration or reflex techniques. If the tachycardia mechanism is abnormal automatism, in addition to the above, these tachycardias are characterized by the fact that they are not induced or interrupted by asynchronous or programmed atrial stimulation, and spontaneous induction does not require a delay in intraatrial or nodal conduction [21–23]. Atrial tachycardias based on abnormal automaticity are often characterized by the so-called "warm-up" phenomenon (gradual shortening of the tachycardia cycle length with each successive complex).

The characteristic features of atrial tachycardias based on a trigger mechanism are an increase in the cycle length of the tachycardia followed by its cessation; the initial cycle length of the tachycardia is equal to the cycle length of the asynchronous stimulation or the value of the coupling interval of the programmed extrastimulus; asynchronous or programmed atrial stimulation may induce (interrupt) or have no effect on the tachycardia.

The peculiarities of intra-atrial tachycardias that distinguish them from AVRT are that the start of intra-atrial tachycardia occurs after conduction delay in the atria, whereas in AVRT, conduction delay occurs after conduction delay in the His-Purkinje system [24]. Intra-atrial tachycardias, unlike AVRT, are generally not provoked by ventricular stimulation. Moreover, the very existence of an intra-atrial tachycardia whose loop of re-entry involves ventricular structures is improbable.

5. Catheter ablation of accessory pathways in WPW syndrome

Nowadays, due to relative safety and high efficiency, the technique of radiofrequency catheter ablation (RFCA) of APs in the treatment of patients with WPW syndrome, even with minimal disease symptoms, has become widespread. The indications for RFCA in patients with WPW developed by the 2019 ESC Guidelines for the Management of Patients with supraventricular tachycardia" are used in everyday clinical practice [18]. In fact, RFCA is a method of choice in patients with WPW.

5.1 Mapping technique for AP topic initialization

Determination of the area of interest for the effective RF application is based on the data of activation mapping, which verifies the area where the elimination of APs conduction is most likely to occur during RF application. APs mapping is performed on the sinus rhythm (possible only in manifest WPW syndrome), asynchronous ventricular and/or atrial stimulation, as well as on AVRT background [25–27]. The key point for determining the point of effective radiofrequency application is the simultaneous registration of bipolar and unipolar signals from the ablation electrode.

5.2 Using of 3D cardiac mapping system for accessory pathway ablation

Advanced 3D cardiac mapping systems are commonly used to detect and ablate regular APs located in AV rings. Modern 3D mapping systems like Carto, NAVX, and Rhythmia have several advantages in treating complex arrhythmias. These are activation mapping with a 3D mapping system that allows accurate catheter location and facilitates the identification of the ablated target. In addition, the 3D mapping system can reconstruct detailed 3D surface anatomy of structures and catheter markings in real-time virtual space.

Previous studies have shown that the 3D cardiac mapping approach significantly reduces fluoroscopic exposure time but does not increase the probability of acute success of supraventricular tachycardia ablation [28, 29]. However, some recent studies have found that the 3D mapping technique had a significantly higher acute success rate and lower recurrence rate than the standard technique in patients with posterior septal APs associated with CS diverticulum. In addition, fluoroscopy time and procedure time were also significantly reduced while using the 3D mapping system method. These results are consistent with previous studies that demonstrated the efficacy and 3D mapping system method safety in the ablation of various APs types [30, 31]. Therefore, the 3D mapping method had more benefits for these patients with posterior septal APs associated with CS diverticulum, as no recurrence and no complications were observed in patients under 3D mapping method control at follow-up.

5.3 RFCA performing

Both conventional and irrigated electrodes can be used to perform RFCA of APs. The following parameters of RFCA are applied: average power –40 ± 10 W, average heating temperature – 51 ± 9°C, during conventional ablation electrode. Occasionally, if the actions mentioned above do not lead to effective RFCA of APs, it is reasonable to use irrigated electrodes. Their application is especially relevant for the ablation of septal and right APs, localized in the free wall. As a rule, we use average power parameters of 35 ± 5 W and average temperature parameters of 45 ± 5°C at an irrigation rate of 17 ml/min [15].

Both transaortic (retrograde) and transseptal access can be used for RFCA of left-sided APs.

5.4 In transaortic positioning

Under X-ray control, the ablation catheter is retrogradely inserted into the left heart and positioned in the area of the APs location - the zone of its optimal mapping on the sinus rhythm (in case of manifest APs), asynchronous or programmed ventricular stimulation (in case of concealed APs) or AVRT background (if the patient can tolerate tachycardia well) (**Figure 10**).

Transseptal access is performed after the transseptal puncture, which is performed under X-ray and transesophageal or intracardiac ultrasound control. After the atrial septal puncture under X-ray control, an ablation electrode is positioned into the area of interest in the left atrium via a long introducer.

Figure 11 illustrates the position of the ablation electrode inserted into the left atrium using a transseptal approach for the left anterior localization of AP.

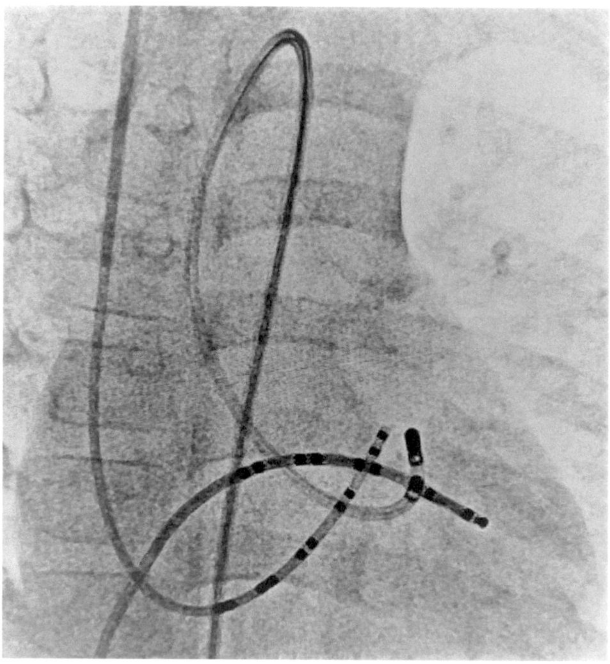

Figure 10.
Transaortic (retrograde) placement of an ablation catheter into the left ventricle where the AP is located.

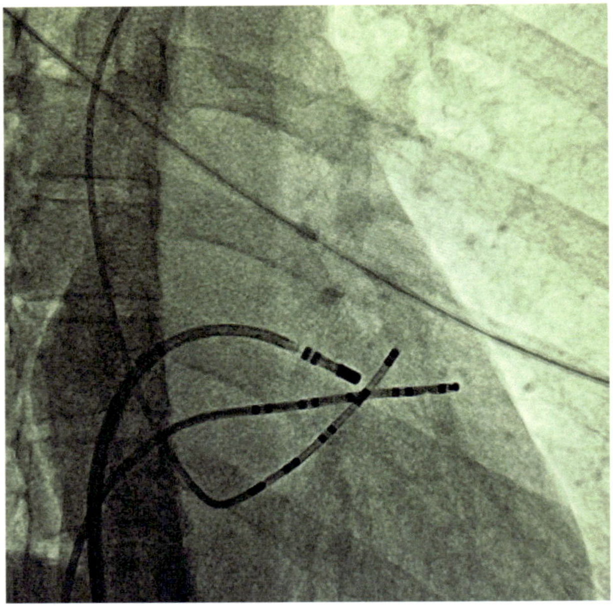

Figure 11.
Transseptal catheter access into the left atrium for ablation of left side located AP.

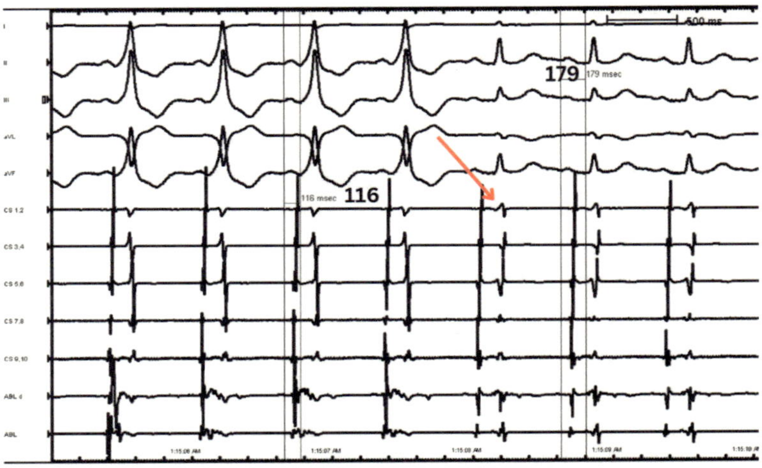

Figure 12.
Ablation effect during the procedure: The AP is closed; the impulse passes through the AV conduction (indicated by the arrow). P-R was 116 ms, after ablation prolonged to 179 ms.

When the optimal positioning and stabilization of the ablation catheter in the point of interest is achieved during RF exposure on the sinus rhythm background, conduction elimination along the APs is noted (**Figure 12**).

Upon successful RF treatment of the concealed left lateral APs during ventricular stimulation, a change in the type of retrograde atrial activation from eccentric to central type is observed (**Figure 13**).

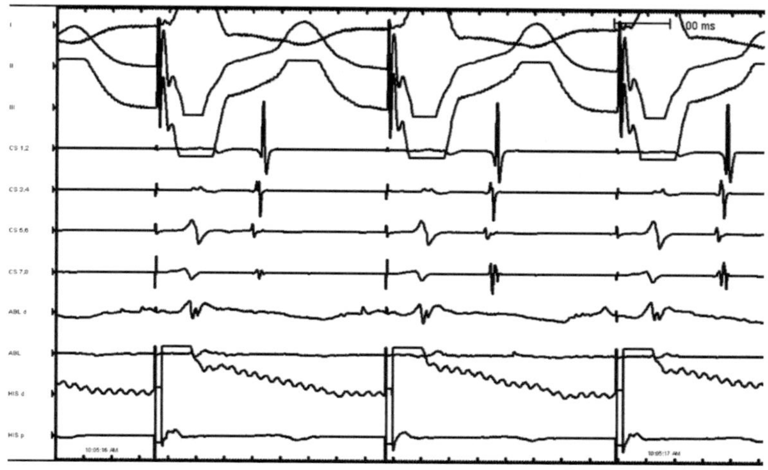

Figure 13.
One of the criteria for the effectiveness of ablation with retrograde stimulation is that the conduction along the AP is stopped, and retrograde atrial activation changes from eccentric to central type.

In certain cases, V-A dissociation, detected during asynchronous ventricular stimulation, is a sign of effective APs elimination.

5.5 Evaluation of RFCA efficacy

A repeated EP studies protocol is performed to assess efficacy, confirming persistent conduction elimination by APs (absence of AVRT induction, presence or absence of VA -conduction - VA dissociation, change in geometry to a central type of atrial retrograde activation (**Figures 12** and **13**).

The operation is considered successful after intravenous administration of 1 ml of 0.1% atropine sulphate solution during the control protocol of EP studies and a waiting period approaching 30 minutes [32].

5.6 Cryotherapy in the ablation of tachycardias associated with APs

Catheter-based cryotherapy has been introduced for the treatment of various arrhythmia types. The main advantage of using cryoenergy is to avoid the formation of useless and undesirable lesions by cryomapping [33]. Cryomapping allows an accurate map of a needed region in advance. This aspect of cryoenergetics may help to reduce the risk of AV node damage. In addition, catheter adhesion ("cryoadhesion") to cardiac tissue prevents the catheter tip displacement or sliding motion during lesion formation seen with radiofrequency energy application [34].

Recent studies have demonstrated the safety of the cryoablation system in terms of preventing damage to the compact AV node. It should be pointed out that the tip size of the cryoablation catheter varied in different studies. Khairy et al. reported that a cryocatheter with a more extended electrode tip could cause larger lesions of equal depth according to a comparative study using a cryocatheter with a tip of 4, 6, and 8 mm [35]. The 8 mm tip cryocatheter may provide a higher success rate, but it may increase the incidence of adverse events by creating larger lesions that may reach the compact AV node.

5.7 Complications associated with RFCA of APs

Currently, complications during endocardial EP studies and RFCA of APs can be divided into three groups:

- complications associated with a puncture and catheterization of vessels (haematoma, deep vein thrombosis, marginal damage of the femoral artery wall, arteriovenous fistula, and pneumothorax);
- complications during catheter manipulations (heart valve damage, microembolism, perforation of myocardial wall or coronary sinus, dissection of coronary sinus, and its thrombosis);
- complications caused by RF exposure (AV blockade of various degrees, myocardial perforation, spasm or occlusion of coronary arteries, transient cerebral circulatory disturbance, and other cerebrovascular complications).

Author details

Adil Baimbetov
Interventional Cardiology and Arrhythmology Department, Syzganov' National Scientific Centre of Surgery, Almaty, Kazakhstan

*Address all correspondence to: kazpace@gmail.com

References

[1] Di Biase L, Gianni C, Bagliani G, Padeletti L. Arrhythmias involving the atrioventricular junction. Cardiac Electrophysiology Clinics. 2017;**9**(3):435-452. DOI: 10.1016/j.ccep.2017.05.004

[2] Becker AE, Anderson RH, Durrer D, et al. The anatomical substrate of WPW syndrome: A clinicopathologic correlation in patients. Circulation. 1978;**57**:870-879

[3] Leonelli FM, De Ponti R, Bagliani G. Arrhythmias with bystander accessory pathways. Cardiac Electrophysiology Clinics. 2020;**12**(4):495-503. Epub 2020 Oct 12. DOI: 10.1016/j.ccep.2020.08.009

[4] Hanna Deschamps E, Hanna EB. Atrioventricular accessory pathways: Mechanisms, electrocardiograms, and associated arrhythmias. Southern Medical Journal. 2016;**109**(10):670-676. DOI: 10.14423

[5] Jastrzebski M, Pitak M, Rudzinski A, Czarnecka D. Wide QRS complex tachycardia in a patient with concealed accessory pathway: What is the mechanism? Journal of Cardiovascular Electrophysiology. 2016;**27**(9):1121-1123. Epub 2016 May 12. DOI: 10.1111/jce.12992

[6] Gonzalez JE, Zipse MM, Nguyen DT, Sauer WH. Antidromic atrioventricular reciprocating tachycardia using a concealed retrograde conducting left lateral accessory pathway. Cardiac Electrophysiology Clinics. 2016;**8**(1):37-43. Epub 2016 Jan 11. DOI: 10.1016/j.ccep.2015.10.001

[7] Nayfeh M, Refaat MM. Is there a need for a novel algorithm for accessory pathways localization? Journal of Cardiovascular Electrophysiology. 2022;**33**(5):962-965. Epub 2022 Feb 26. DOI: 10.1111/jce.15414

[8] Baek SM, Song MK, Uhm JS, Kim GB, Bae EJ. New algorithm for accessory pathway localization focused on screening septal pathways in pediatric patients with Wolff-Parkinson-white syndrome. Heart Rhythm. 2020;**17**(12):2172-2179. Epub 2020 Jul 16. DOI: 10.1016/j.hrthm.2020.07.016

[9] Crinion D, Baranchuk A. Algorithms to identify accessory Pathways' location on the 12-Lead electrocardiogram. Cardiac Electrophysiology Clinics. 2020;**12**(4):465-474. Epub 2020 Oct 9. DOI: 10.1016/j.ccep.2020.08.007

[10] Arruda MS, McClelland JH. Wang X, et al/development and validation of an ECG algorithm for identifying accessory pathway ablation site in Wolff-Parkinson-white syndrome. Journal of Cardiovascular Electrophysiology. 1998;**9**:2-12

[11] Peters NS, Rowland E, Bennett JG, et al. The Wolff-Parkinson-white syndrome: The cellular substrate for conduction in the accessory atrioventricular pathway. European Heart Journal. 1994;**15**:98

[12] Ho SY. Accessory atrioventricular pathways: Getting to the origins. Circulation. 2008;**117**:1502-1504

[13] Bhatia A, Sra J, Akhtar M. Preexcitation syndromes. Current Problems in Cardiology. 2016;**41**(3):99-137. DOI: 10.1016/j.cpcardiol.2015.11.002

[14] Haissaguerre M, Gaita F, Marcus FI, Clementy J. Radiofrequency catheter ablation of accessory pathways. A contemporary review. Journal of

Cardiovascular Electrophysiology. 1994;**5**:532-552

[15] Baimbetov AK, Bizhanov KA, Sagatov IE, et al. Outcomes of catheter treatment for patients with WPW syndrome: Single center experience. Bulletin of Surgery in Kazakhstan. 2017;**4**(53):5-10

[16] Ali R, Tahir A, Nadeem M, et al. / Antidromic atrioventricular reentry tachycardia with Wolff Parkinson white syndrome: A rare beast. Cureus. 2018;**10**(5):e2642. DOI: 10.7759/cureus.2642

[17] Corcia MCG, Stuart G, Walsh M, et al. /redo accessory pathway ablation in the pediatric population. Journal of Interventional Cardiac Electrophysiology. 2022;**63**(3):639-649. Epub 2021 Nov 22. DOI: 10.1007/s10840-021-01064-1

[18] Brugada J, Katritsis DG, Arbelo E, et al. ESC scientific document group. ESC guidelines for the management of patients with supraventricular tachycardia the task force for the management of patients with supraventricular tachycardia of the European Society of Cardiology (ESC). European Heart Journal. 2020;**41**:655-720

[19] Page RL, Joglar JA, Caldwell MA, et al. Evidence review committee chair. 2015 ACC/AHA/HRS guideline for the Management of Adult Patients with Supraventricular Tachycardia: A report of the American College of Cardiology/American Heart Association task force on clinical practice guidelines and the Heart Rhythm Society. Circulation. 2016;**133**:e506-e574. Erratum in: Circulation. 2016;134:e234-5

[20] Josephson ME. Josephson's Clinical Cardiac Electrophysiology: Techniques and Interpretations. 4th ed. Philadelphia: Wolters Kluwer; 2015

[21] Nakagawa H, Lazzara R, Jackman WM. Development and validation of an ECG algorithm for identifying accessory pathway ablation site in Wolff-Parkinson-white syndrome. Journal of Cardiovascular Electrophysiology. 1998;**9**:2-12

[22] Schricker AA, Winkle R, Moskovitz R, et al. Open-window mapping of accessory pathways utilizing high-density mapping. Journal of Interventional Cardiac Electrophysiology. 2021;**61**:525-533

[23] Campbell RM, Strieper MJ, Frias P. A., et al/survey of current practice of pediatric electrophysiologists for asymptomatic Wolff-Parkinson-white syndrome. Pediatrics. 2003;**111**(3):e245-e247. DOI: 10.1542/peds.111.3.e245

[24] Pappone C, Santinelli V, Rosanio S, et al. Usefulness of invasive electrophysiologic testing to stratify the risk of arrhythmic events in asymptomatic patients with Wolff-Parkinson-white pattern. Journal of the American College of Cardiology. 2003;**41**(2):239-244. DOI: 10.1016/s0735-1097(02)02706-7

[25] Bar-Cohen Y, Cecchin F, Alexander ME, et al. Cryoablation for accessory pathways located near normal conduction tissues or within the coronary venous system in children and young adults. Heart Rhythm. 2006;**3**:253-258

[26] Huang H, Wang X, Ouyang F, Antz M. Catheter ablation of anteroseptal accessory pathway in the non-coronary aortic sinus. Europace. 2006;**8**:1041-1044

[27] Xu G, Liu T. Liu E, et al/ radiofrequency catheter ablation at the

non-coronary cusp for the treatment of Para-hisian accessory pathways. Europace. 2015;**17**:962-968. DOI: 10.1093/europace/euu271

[28] Mah DY, Miyake CY, Sherwin ED, et al. The use of an integrated electroanatomic mapping system and intracardiac echocardiography to reduce radiation exposure in children and young adults undergoing ablation of supraventricular tachycardia. Europace. 2014;**16**(2):277-283

[29] Stec S, Śledź J, Mazij M, et al. Feasibility of implementation of a "simplified, No-X-ray, no-lead apron, two-catheter approach" for ablation of supraventricular arrhythmias in children and adults. Journal of Cardiovascular Electrophysiology. 2014;**25**(8):866-874

[30] Bergonti M, Dello Russo A, Sicuso R, Ribatti V, Compagnucci P, Catto V, et al. Long-term outcomes of near-zero radiation ablation of paroxysmal supraventricular tachycardia: A comparison with fluoroscopy-guided approach. JACC: Clinical Electrophysiology. 2021;**7**(9):1108-1117

[31] Mah DY, Miyake CY, Elizabeth D. Sherwin, et al/the use of an integrated electroanatomic mapping system and intracardiac echocardiography to reduce radiation exposure in children and young adults undergoing ablation of supraventricular tachycardia. EP Europace. 2014;**16**(2):277-283

[32] Nakagawa H, Jackman WM. Catheter ablation of paroxysmal supraventricular tachycardia. Circulation. 2007;**116**:2465-2428

[33] Karadeniz C, Akdeniz C, Turan O, Tuzcu V. Cryoablation of septal accessory pathways in children: Midterm results. Pacing and Clinical Electrophysiology. 2014;**37**:1095-1099

[34] Bar-Cohen Y, Cecchin F, Alexander ME, et al. Cryoablation of right-sided accessory pathways in children: Report of efficacy and safety after 10-year experience and follow-up. Europace. 2013;**15**:1651-1656

[35] Khairy P, Rivard L, Guerra PG, et al. Morpho- metric ablation lesion characteristics comparing 4, 6, and 8 mm electrode-tip cryocatheters. Journal of Cardiovascular Electrophysiology. 2008;**19**:1203-1207

Chapter 2

Experimental and Computational Models of Atrial Fibrillation

Rafael J. Ramirez, Samuel J. Bergman and Jamal A. Masri

Abstract

Atrial fibrillation (AF) is the most common cardiac arrhythmia with potentially severe consequences that include stroke and sudden death. A high prevalence in the general population, combined with severe morbidity and mortality, make AF a major public health concern. Factors that predispose to AF are numerous and complex and include electrical, structural, neurohumoral, immunological and inflammatory remodeling of the heart. This chapter provides a review of animal and computational models of AF that have provided insights into this complex arrhythmia. These models bridge the gap between nonclinical and clinical research, and have been indispensable for expanding our understanding of the many factors that contribute to progression of this arrhythmia. Using a wide variety of investigational approaches and scientific models, researchers gain insights into mechanisms that affect the onset and progression of AF, as well as test novel treatments and therapeutic strategies.

Keywords: atrial fibrillation, experimental animal models, computational models, arrhythmia, cardiac electrophysiology

1. Introduction

Atrial Fibrillation (AF) is the most common sustained arrhythmia that is linked with negative health outcomes [1]. The Global Burden project estimated that in 2016, about 46.3 million people globally were affected by AF [2]. In 2004, the lifetime risk of developing AF for white men and women over 40 years was about 1 in 4 [3]. However, a decade later, this risk increased to approximately 1 in 3 for white individuals and 1 in 5 for Black individuals [4]. In the United States, between 3 and 6 million individuals currently suffer from AF, and predictions suggest this could rise to approximately 6 to 16 million by 2050 [5, 6]. Meanwhile, in Europe there were about 9 million cases of AF in 2010 among those aged 55 and older. This number is anticipated to grow to 14 million by 2060 [7, 8]. Projections for Asia suggest that by 2050, AF will be diagnosed in roughly 72 million people, with almost 3 million of those experiencing AF-related strokes [9, 10]. The clinical risk factors for AF include advancing age, diabetes, hypertension, congestive heart failure, rheumatic and nonrheumatic valve disease, and myocardial infarction [11].

This chapter reviews different types of large and small animal models of AF that have been developed as investigational tools for the study of mechanisms and treatments of AF. This review includes the development of computational models that have provided further insights that are often untestable in animal model experimentation.

2. Sterile pericarditis-induced AF

Sterile pericarditis emerged as an early, valuable approach for inducing AF in animal models. This model involves the introduction of irritants into the pericardial space, triggering a localized inflammatory response that alters atrial conduction and refractoriness, favoring a substrate for AF initiation and persistence. Several techniques have been utilized to induce sterile pericarditis, each having distinct aspects of the inflammatory response and overall development of AF.

2.1 Techniques to elicit sterile pericarditis

Mineral Oil Injection: The injection of sterile mineral oil into the pericardial space serves as an effective technique to induce sterile pericarditis. This method triggers an inflammatory response characterized by immune cell infiltration and cytokine release, resulting in an environment conducive to AF-associated inflammation.

Talc Administration: Intrapericardial talc injection induces inflammation via pleuropericardial irritation, leading to fibrinous pericarditis. The resulting inflammatory cascade extends to the atrial myocardium, promoting electrophysiological changes comparable of those seen in clinical AF.

Lipopolysaccharide (LPS) Administration: LPS is a component of Gram-negative bacterial cell walls. When it is introduced intrapericardially, it elicits an immune response similar to infection-induced pericarditis. This approach demonstrates the role of immune activation in AF pathogenesis, offering insights into the connection between inflammation and arrhythmogenesis.

When creating an animal model of AF, there are a variety of techniques employed to create a suitable inflammatory response that is conducive to formation of a pro-fibrillatory substrate. Sterile pericarditis created in a swine model has been achieved by placing double-layer gauze on the surface of the left and right atrial walls, combined with spreading talcum powder on the exterior of atrial surfaces [12]. A similar approach for inducing AF in a canine model using sterile pericarditis employed talcum powder coating, followed by single-layer gauze placement on the right and left atrial free walls, which was adequate for creating an atrial substrate prone to AF [13]. Another approach employing sterile pericarditis in canines used arachidonic acid applied to atrial appendages to trigger an acute inflammatory response promoting AF, where treatment with anti-inflammatory drugs attenuated arrhythmogenic effects [14]. Furthermore, simple pericardiotomies, involving a cutdown of the pericardium, have been performed on rabbits to induce AF. Here, histone deacetylase (HDAC), an epigenetic regulator of cardiac remodeling during cardiovascular disease, was inhibited to reduce instances of AF in rabbits [15]. Within these models, researchers have observed increased frequency of premature atrial contractions, shortened atrial refractory periods, cardiac hypertrophy and elevated fibrosis that is commonly observed in clinical cases of AF [12, 13, 15].

2.2 Large animal models utilizing sterile pericarditis

Sterile pericarditis-induced AF has been primarily explored in larger animal models like dogs, pigs and goats, as they share a comparable atrial anatomy and size to humans. Large animal models allow for the introduction of catheter-based electrophysiological mapping and monitoring, making them suitable for studying mechanisms of AF [16, 17]. This feature of large animal models makes them useful for studying the spatiotemporal dynamics of AF [14], and offers insights into AF progression from paroxysmal to persistent [18], allowing researchers to investigate mechanisms of reentrant circuits and rotor formation [19–21] that are hallmarks of AF. The utility of the large animal AF model lies in its similarity to human clinical AF, including the ability to maintain high-frequency atrial activation, electrophysiological heterogeneity, electrical remodeling, and reentrant circuit establishment as the principal driver of AF.

Sterile pericarditis as a method for AF induction gives rise to structural and electrical remodeling that is similar to that observed in clinical AF. Characteristics of cardiac remodeling that favor an atrial substrate conducive to AF include persistence of atrial flutter, altered gap junction connexin 40 and 43 distribution, unstable re-entrant circuits near and around the pulmonary veins and atrial septum, presence of short-lived rotors, and a dysregulated inflammatory response [14, 22–26]. These characteristics provide researchers with a reliable and robust environment to study the onset and progression of AF as well as novel treatments that may reduce re-entrant events or mitigate progression of the arrhythmia.

2.3 Insights and implications

Researchers employing sterile pericarditis-induced AF models have investigated the relationship between inflammation, structural remodeling, and electrophysiological changes in the pathogenesis of AF [12, 13, 15, 23, 27]. Through these models, researchers have been able to understand the contributions of pro-inflammatory cytokines, immune cell infiltration, and fibrotic changes to atrial electrical remodeling [15, 23]. These models confirm that inflammation plays a crucial role in creating an arrhythmogenic substrate, and that atrial fibrosis is a critical factor contributing to AF maintenance [15, 27, 28]. Insights from sterile pericarditis models have shaped the development of anti-inflammatory and antifibrotic therapeutic strategies that address underlying mechanisms that drive AF [15].

The use of sterile pericarditis in animal models allows researchers to study the effects of post-operative atrial fibrillation (POAF), a condition that occurs in 30–50% of patients several days following open heart surgery who have no prior medical history of AF [29, 30]. Other studies have claimed these occurrences for POAF to range from 10 to 65% of patients, where onset of AF occurred around 2–3 days following surgery [31]. Observing and studying inflammatory mechanisms in controlled instances of POAF has been done through inducing sterile pericarditis in canine and swine models as they share comparative structural anatomies and electrophysiological properties to that of a human heart [12, 13, 27]. Open heart surgery leading to AF can lead to a multitude of complications that compromise cardiac functionality. Heightened risk of myocardial ischemia, decreased diastolic filling and cardiac output, loss of optimal atrial contraction leading to increased pulmonary arterial pressure make up several of these complications [32]. As a result, POAF is associated with increased stroke risk, mortality, and hospital stays [31, 33]. Developing novel treatments to reduce the risks exacerbated by AF drives much of the current research, making animal models an indispensable research approach. Sterile pericarditis provides a reliable and replicable model to assess onset, progression, maintenance, and treatment of AF.

3. Canine models of AF

3.1 Inducing AF in canine models

The research behind canine models of AF unravels a range of techniques designed to replicate the intricate arrhythmic behavior that can be observed in humans. These methods provide insights into distinct features of AF pathophysiology. One of the most common and efficacious techniques in inducing AF in canine models involves rapid atrial pacing (tachypacing), a technique that simulates the electrophysiological dynamics of AF through sustained high-frequency stimulation, commonly induced from pacemaker leads extending into the walls of the atrium [34–42]. By subjecting the atria to prolonged episodes of rapid pacing, researchers simulate the conditions that induce atrial electrical and structural remodeling similar to the AF substrate. This approach provides a model that recapitulates irregular atrial activation observed in clinical AF, but also shows conduction pathways and refractory period alterations associated with AF onset and stabilization.

In addition to rapid atrial pacing, atrial remodeling induced by heart failure serves as an avenue to understand the relationship between structural and electrical changes leading to AF. Studies have revealed that heart failure triggers substantial atrial remodeling, involving changes in ion channel expression, action potential characteristics, and conduction properties [41, 43]. These changes set the stage for the initiation and perpetuation of AF, further emphasizing how the nature of AF arrhythmogenesis may not all be entirely the same.

3.2 Electrophysiological insights and mapping

Electrophysiological exploration in canine models has ushered in an increased understanding of the mechanisms at play that govern induction and persistence of atrial fibrillation. By carefully mapping and monitoring the electrical landscape of the atria in these models, researchers have expanded their understanding of the initiation and maintenance of AF. Among these insights, atrial refractoriness dispersion takes center stage, demonstrating the critical role it plays in creating a conducive substrate for rotors and reentrant circuits, the hallmark of AF. The canine model's fidelity to human atrial physiology allows researchers to uncover variations in refractoriness across different atrial regions, providing a greater understanding of the arrhythmia's onset and persistence.

Conduction velocity alterations also emerge as a key characteristic in AF, clarifying how variations in atrial conduction contribute to the irregular rhythm. Canine AF models have shed light on the regional disparities in conduction velocity, depicting the complex conduction pathways that facilitate the chaotic activation patterns characteristic of AF. These observations not only deepen our understanding of AF but also give rise to potential targets for therapeutics aimed at normalizing conduction velocity and restoring atrial rhythm within patients experiencing AF.

The current understanding of electrophysiological remodeling has been advanced with application of high-resolution electrophysiological mapping techniques, such as the use of catheter-based mapping, in canine models. By employing these techniques, researchers can visualize activation patterns during AF, and further understand the spatial heterogeneity of atrial activation. The atrial dimensions in dogs, similar to those in humans, allow for accurate representation of conduction pathways and provide for the identification of regions prone to reentry. This approach enables scientists to precisely map the pathways through which AF perpetuates, guiding the development of therapeutic strategies that target specific regions of interest.

3.3 Translational implications of canine AF models

Translational implications of canine models in AF research extend far beyond the laboratory, holding promise in shaping clinical interventions and management strategies for individuals experiencing more severe cases of AF. These models not only unveil the dynamic mechanisms underlying onset and persistence of AF, but also serve as testing grounds for novel therapeutic interventions. Using canine models in AF exploration can pave the way for innovative strategies that have a meaningful and effective impact on clinical care. Insights from canine models have been instrumental in refining catheter ablation techniques, which serves as a popular and common practice in treating AF and in AF management. Through accurately mapping conduction pathways and visualizing reentrant circuits [21], these models contribute to the advancement of ablation strategies, leading to improved success rates and patient outcomes.

Furthermore, canine models facilitate the evaluation of antiarrhythmic drugs, bridging the gap between experimental findings and clinical translation. Through these models, researchers can assess the efficacy and safety of potential therapeutic agents, steering drug development towards more targeted and effective treatments for AF [35, 43]. The canine model's ability to simulate the dynamic environment of AF enhances the predictive value of preclinical trials, ensuring that only the most promising candidates proceed to human trials, thus expediting the drug discovery process. By serving as a bridge for translational research, canine models ultimately increase the tools available for clinicians to combat this arrhythmia in patient settings.

Spontaneous AF is a condition that has been observed to naturally occur in dogs and has been shown to have linkage to certain heart diseases, such as myxomatous mitral valve disease. This dysfunction can lead to enlargement of the left atrium and overall, heart failure, a prognosis commonly seen in clinical cases, increasing mortality [44, 45]. Canine models have seen high use in studying electrophysiological implications of AF. In canine models of AF, action potential durations in pulmonary veins are notably shorter than the surrounding left atrium, having an altered resting membrane potential and lower inward rectifier (I_{K1}) current density [46–48]. Induction of AF in dogs has been mostly achieved by atrial tachypacing [34–42], sometimes following catheter-induced atrioventricular node ablation to separate the electrical connection between the atria and ventricles [49]. Notably, atrial tachypacing does not always lead to sustained episodes of AF in dogs: one study found that to achieve sustained AF (AF episodes lasting >15 minutes), atrial tachypacing at a rate of 400 bpm was needed over a 6-week time period [42]. In this model, the resultant decreased atrial refractory period and slowed conduction velocity was directly correlated with how long animal subjects were exposed to atrial tachypacing [42]. Additionally, inflammatory models, such as sterile pericarditis-induced AF, has emerged as a widely used model in studying AF, as outlined above. These models helped reveal the presence of short-lived rotors during episodes of AF as well as demonstrating a correlation between post operative AF and heterogenous atrial conduction [14, 26, 27].

Canine models of AF have shed light on the relationship between the autonomic nervous system and induction of AF. Canine models experiencing atrial tachypacing showed inducibility of AF to be significantly decreased by sympathovagal denervation, indicating that the triggering and modulation of AF episodes lasting at least 1 hour could be related to sympathovagal stimulation [50, 51]. One study found both isoproterenol and acetylcholine were useful in inducing AF and prolonging AF duration [52]. Indeed, combining autonomic stimulation with atrial tachypacing has been proven a reliable trigger for AF in canine models, with acute episodes lasting more than 1 hour [53].

Atrial remodeling in humans, to a degree that is conducive to AF, can occur secondarily to ventricular remodeling [54]. Ventricular tachypacing models of heart failure in canines have been used to study atrial remodeling, where alterations of connexins, reduced expression of ionic currents including I_{CaL}, I_{to}, and I_{Ks}, and increased expression of Na-Ca exchanger activity (I_{NCX}), has been observed [41, 55]. These changes parallel various types of cellular remodeling observed in human cardiomyocytes, allowing ventricular tachypacing in canine models to serve as a suitable example for studying AF [56].

Canine models have provided a fruitful platform to study mechanisms, progression, and treatments for various arrhythmias, AF in particular. Nevertheless, canine models do come with limitations. Genetic heterogeneity, stemming from the use of different dog breeds, poses challenges to assessing and studying genetic differences between healthy and AF states in dogs as well as comparing them to human cases. Dog breeds need to be selected and monitored when choosing how the model will be created. Additionally, there are differences in coronary collateralization, heart weight-to-body weight ratio, and ECG metrics (P waves, QRS complexes, and QT intervals) compared to humans [57]. Nonetheless, canines have provided a fruitful model for studying AF.

4. Goat models of AF

In the realm of atrial fibrillation research, the goat model stands out as particularly insightful. Goats can sustain AF for extended periods, up to several weeks. This longitudinal property renders them invaluable in observing long-term structural and electrical modifications that persistent AF induces. However, no model is without its limitations. In the case of goats, researchers must grapple with issues like pronounced ECG variability, characteristically shorter action potentials, a predominance of the left-sided coronary system, and a scarcity of detailed cellular electrophysiological data.

4.1 Atrial tachypaced goat model

Most goat models of AF have employed an atrial tachypacing (ATP) approach that was pioneered by Wijffels [58–61]. The model design involved surgical thoracotomy, where electrodes were meticulously placed on atrial epicardial surfaces. Goats were treated with a regimen of ampicillin to ward off infections and buprenorphine to manage pain. After recovery, goats were instrumented with an external fibrillation pacemaker. This was achieved using a suspended cable connected to an electrode positioned on the goat's neck, which interfaced with a multi-channel monitoring apparatus. This design ensured goats retained their full range of movement. Pacemaker operations were managed automatically by computer software, designed to distinguish sinus rhythms from atrial fibrillation.

Any detection of regular sinus rhythm immediately triggered the software to deliver biphasic stimuli, thus re-inducing AF.

4.2 Properties of atrial tachypacing goat AF models

Observations from the tachypaced Goat Models unveiled intriguing patterns. The onset of AF initiated a period of electrical remodeling within the first 24 hours. Tachypacing had a pronounced impact on repolarization and atrial excitability. Initial AF episodes were fleeting, often concluding within seconds. But over time, these episodes began to prolong in duration—lasting roughly 20 seconds after a day and then extending into chronic episodes in the weeks that followed. These observations gave rise to the expression, "Atrial Fibrillation Begets Atrial Fibrillation" [60]. As these episodes extended, there was a distinct rise in the fibrillation rate, accompanied by a decrease in the prominence of high-amplitude deflections, making way for more fragmented electrograms.

4.3 Atrial fibrillation begets atrial fibrillation

The concept that AF begets AF was conceived in these early observations [60]. The continual occurrence of AF instigates transformative changes in the heart's structural anatomy and its electrical properties, thereby predisposing it to further AF episodes. In other words, the more frequently, or the longer one experiences AF, the higher the chances of its recurrence and the longer its duration in subsequent events. This cyclical nature of AF poses two primary challenges:

a. Electrical Remodeling: Prolonged AF episodes instigate modifications in ion channel expression in atrial cells. This remodeling can drastically alter a fibrillating heart's response to antiarrhythmic medications, potentially undermining the effectiveness of chemical cardioversion.

b. Rate Adaptation: When transitioning from AF back to sinus rhythm, there's a marked shift in atrial interbeat intervals. An inappropriately adjusted, or even counteractive adaptation of the atrial refractory period can leave the atria vulnerable, escalating the risk of a rapid return to AF.

5. Sheep chronic and acute models of AF

Sheep, as experimental subjects, have proven to be instrumental in the elucidation of AF mechanics. While naturally occurring, AF in sheep is elusive, and multiple ovine model systems have been tailored to mimic the various elements of human AF. These intricate models dive deep, shedding light on the structural, metabolic, and cellular metamorphoses that herald the advent of AF.

5.1 Sheep AF induction by rapid pacing and acetylcholine

Utilizing an *ex vivo* sheep heart protocol, the interplay of rapid pacing and acetylcholine in acute AF genesis has been extensively studied [19, 20, 62–65]. Organ harvest is performed under deep anesthesia using pentobarbital. Hearts are surgically removed and swiftly immersed in cold cardioplegic solution to preserve their structural and functional integrity. Hearts are then perfused in a Langendorff apparatus, a long-established tool in cardiac research, for further electrical or optical mapping experiments. The coronary arteries are supplied with warm, oxygenated Tyrode's solution at a constant rate, delivered retrogradely through an aortic cannula. AF is then initiated by burst pacing in tandem with acetylcholine or cholinomimetics.

5.2 Sheep AF modulation by interatrial pressure

In this method, the heart is Langendorff perfused with Tyrode's solution. Increasing interatrial pressure by elevating perfusion pressure renders the hearts more susceptible to AF, creating stretch-related AF in sheep hearts [19, 20, 62–64]. The interatrial septum is perforated to equilibrate left and right interatrial pressures (IAP) and venous orifices are ligated to maintain a closed pressure system. Changes in IAP are controlled by adjusting the height of pressure relief outflow tubing with respect to height of the perfused heart. Enhanced inducibility of AF with stretch is reversible, returning to sinus rhythm when IAP is returned to normal physiologic pressures. This stretch-related sheep AF model has been used to explore atrial regions of high rate activity [62–64], differences between acute stretch AF and persistent AF [20], and mechanisms of AF rate acceleration [19].

5.3 Sheep AF induction by intermittent tachypacing

The tachypaced sheep model has offered significant insights into mechanisms of AF. In the intermittent right atrial tachypacing model, sheep are instrumented with a modified pacemaker to deliver a short burst of high frequency (20 Hz) atrial stimulation whenever sinus rhythm is detected [18, 20, 66–69]. In this model, AF progresses from brief runs of AF to long-standing persistent AF which remains self-sustained (in the absence of device tachypacing) for periods as long as 1 year [18]. This progression of AF is characterized by hallmark electrical remodeling, including altered current densities of calcium, sodium and potassium currents; as well as features of structural remodeling including increased fibrosis, cellular hypertrophy, and atrial chamber dilation [18, 67–69]. The dynamic and biophysical properties of AF induced by tachypacing varies with the duration of arrhythmia burden [18], and are distinct from those induced acutely by increased chamber pressure and stretch [20]. This indicates that AF likely represents a broad spectrum of arrhythmia substrates that might not benefit from a single therapeutic approach.

In similar studies, sheep were implanted with dual pacemakers that affected both atrial and ventricular functions using a transvenous approach. A neurostimulator was embedded subcutaneously in the neck region, ensuring rapid atrial pacing capabilities. After post-operative recovery, atrial pacing was initiated at 15 Hz, laying a foundation for persistent AF, with occasional pauses in pacing to ensure accurate rhythm evaluations. The key indicator for the establishment of persistent AF was when sinus rhythm was consistently absent over consecutive assessments [70]. Electrical remodeling, was evidenced by shortened atrial refractory periods and wavelengths *in vivo*. Parallel *in vitro* studies revealed shortened action potential durations and diminished rate adaptation responses. As observed across other large animal AF models, persistent AF wasn't merely an electrical phenomenon, but was paralleled by extensive structural remodeling including atrial enlargement and fibrosis.

6. Rodent models of AF

When diving into the field of AF, murine models stand as key players in providing genetic insights, wide ranges of induction strategies, molecular pathways, cellular remodeling, and targeted interventions. Despite their distinct atrial characteristics compared to humans, mice and rats serve as more-than suitable organisms for understanding the complexities of AF initiation and progression. Central to this exploration is the creation of AF models, a process with an array of techniques that mirror the genetic and structural alterations seen in clinical AF cases. These models allow researchers to investigate intricacies of genetic predispositions, molecular pathways, and electrophysiological changes that culminate in AF.

The use of small animals, such as mice and rats have provided a model for studying AF that is generally both time- and cost-efficient. Given that rodents have smaller hearts compared to humans and other large animal model counterparts, these hearts are more prone to recovering from cases of induced and spontaneous AF. Early on, this observation gave rise to the "critical mass" hypothesis, suggesting smaller animals with smaller hearts were not capable of sustaining a fibrillatory rhythm [71, 72]. This was mainly due to re-entrant circuits not having a large-enough pathway to travel within smaller hearts to sustain fibrillation, as the depolarizing wavefront of the re-entrant circuit would likely collide with the repolarizing tail, stopping fibrillation and restoring homeostatic rhythm. Small animal models require genetic manipulation or programmed electrical stimulation to induce AF, which in some cases only lasts for seconds at a time [57]. Although spontaneous AF is not commonly seen in rodent models, mouse models offer a good platform for studying the AF substrate, rather than the triggers that elicit AF [73]. Nonetheless, there have been several rodent models employed to study characteristics of structural and electrical remodeling seen in clinical AF.

Transesophageal Atrial Pacing Model: Due to low cost and utility of genetic manipulation, rodent models have become the most used animal models in biomedical research. To overcome a lack of spontaneously occurring AF, transesophageal atrial pacing has been used to initiate AF in closed-chest mice and rats [74–79]. A pacing lead is advanced down the esophagus and positioned to capture and stimulate the adjacent atria with burst pacing (as fast as 100 Hz) or programmed premature stimulation. Prolonged transesophageal atrial stimulation increases inducibility of atrial tachyarrhythmias in anesthetized mice, especially in the presence of diminished cell coupling [79], with high reproducibility [78], and particularly in male mice [75]. The summed duration of AF episodes can add up on the order of several minutes for an experimental protocol; however, effects of rapid atrial pacing using a transesophageal approach can be confounded by activation of neighboring nerves and parasympathetic ganglia [75]. Transesophageal atrial pacing has also been used in rat models, where rapid pacing at 83 Hz for 30 seconds induces runs of AF lasting around 10 seconds [74].

Glycolytic Inhibition Model: Rat hearts with glycolytic inhibition display vulnerability to AF in older rats due to Ca^{2+} handling abnormalities. This model underscores the role that glycolysis can play in the development of AF and its relationship with intracellular calcium levels, as the uptake of intracellular Ca^{2+} into the sarcoplasmic reticulum is ATP-dependent. Glycolytic inhibition was induced by adding sodium pyruvate to glucose-free perfusate in isolated rat hearts [80].

Asphyxia Model: This involves burst-pacing and asphyxia in rat models to induce AF. Asphyxia can be induced through clamping of the tracheal tube at the end of an inspiratory cycle. A study researching asphyxia-induced AF in rats found that clamping of the tracheal tube for 35 seconds posed the best time course for inducing AF. Asphyxiation for shorter periods were associated with lowered AF inducibility while longer time periods were associated with prolonged atrioventricular block and severe cases of hypotension [81].

Myocardial Infarction Model: Rats with induced myocardial infarction (MI) through coronary artery ligation can be used to study mechanisms of AF. Although post-infarction rats exhibit remodeling of the extracellular matrix and increased matrix metalloproteinase activity, AF may not always be observable through ECG recordings [82, 83]. These models experience collagen and fibrotic accumulation between atrial cardiomyocytes, conducive to an AF substrate [82, 84].

Spontaneous Hypertension Model: Rats in this model are genetically predisposed to systemic hypertension, displaying increased fibrosis of the left atrium. Activation of the renin-angiotensin system, as a result of hypertension, contributes to progression of a fibrotic substrate. In this model, effective refractory period is unchanged; however, increased fibrosis predisposes to an AF substrate [85, 86].

Dilated Cardiomyopathy Model: Transgenic mice with overexpressed GTPase RhoA, muscle-restricted putative coiled-coil (MURC) protein, and/or tumor necrosis factor-α, replicate aspects of dilated cardiomyopathy. These models display substrates related to AF through increased fibrosis (induced by GTPase RhoA and further stimulated with MURC protein) and downregulated connexin40, revealing a connection between structural changes and onset and progression of AF [87–90].

Hypertrophic Cardiomyopathy Model: Mouse models with accelerated atrial repolarization replicate aspects of hypertrophic cardiomyopathy. Inducing AF in these models has been done through overexpression of junctin, a calsequestrin-binding protein; junctate, a calcium-binding protein associated with the calcium storage capacity within the sarcoplasmic reticulum; GTPase, and Rac1, both regulators of NADPH oxidase activity [91–93]. Prolonged episodes of AF have been observed in rodent models showing overexpression of cardiac Gαq, a mediator of alpha-adrenoceptor, angiotensin II, and endothelin, a protein involved in blood pressure regulation and blood vessel constriction [94]. These models create a substrate for development of AF, drawing a relationship between electrophysiological changes and arrhythmogenesis similar to clinical AF.

In rodents, various models have been employed to induce AF that provide insight into arrhythmia mechanisms. These models capture diverse aspects of the development of AF, highlighting structural changes and electrophysiological abnormalities that contribute to the AF substrate. However, rodent models also come with their own limitations as there are substantial differences in heart scale and electrophysiology between humans and rodents that pose translational research challenges. Rodents have varied action potential morphology and duration attributed to higher resting heart rates, ion channel expression, and current densities [95]. Because of this, tools used to induce AF in large animals, such as catheter-ablations and pacemaker-induced tachycardias have proved difficult to replicate in small animal counterparts [96]. Regardless of these drawbacks, rodent models offer avenues with high potential and value in researching therapeutic interventions.

6.1 Genetic mapping: genetic attributes of AF

Mice and rats serve as laboratories for genetic exploration, enabling us to better understand the genetic landscape of AF. Through genetic manipulations, researchers have a better understanding of how AF originates and persists. Genetic modifications targeting ion channels such as KCNA5, KCNH2, and KCNJ2, as well as calcium handling proteins, such as RyR2 and SERCA2a, offer insights into molecular pathways underlying AF [97, 98]. These genetic manipulations replicate mutations seen clinically, bridging genetic anomalies with molecular conditions that promote arrhythmogenesis.

6.2 Induction of AF in murine models

The induction of AF in murine models has been attributed to diverse strategies, echoing the multitudes of causes that drive the arrhythmogenesis of the clinical condition. While rapid atrial pacing emerges as a prominent approach, simulating the rapid firing characteristic of AF, it's only one technique employed within murine models [99]. Techniques like transesophageal atrial burst pacing over a short period and surgical interventions introduce different AF triggers, providing the arrhythmia's varied nature [75]. Each induction strategy reflects distinct characteristics of AF causation, reflecting the relationship between genetics and triggers that promote its onset.

6.3 Insights from murine models: cellular remodeling

Murine models of AF not only offer insight into genetic and molecular events, but also bring to light the wide array of cellular remodeling that can be observed. These models reflect differences in remodeling patterns encompassing action potential duration changes, altered calcium dynamics, and fibrosis development [100]. Through these changes in cellular remodeling, as a result of variance in gene expression, researchers have been able to better map the pathway of cellular transformations, furthering the understanding underlying molecular cues and genetic predispositions that bring about these changes. By unveiling these patterns, we uncover the pathways in which genetic expression influences cellular remodeling, paving the way for targeted interventions.

6.4 Translational implications of murine models

The murine models' ability to provide insights into AF initiation and persistence extends to targeted interventions, paving the way for laboratory research to guide and influence clinical applications. The combination of genetic manipulation, a wide range of induction strategies, and diverse cellular remodeling helps researchers gain knowledge and direction in the development of interventions and therapeutics that address the diverse characteristics that cause AF. Pharmacological regulation and modulation of ion channels, calcium handling, and anti-inflammatory pathways emerge as promising frontiers in better understanding and treating AF [97, 100]. By targeting specific remodeling pathways, these interventions hold the potential to prevent, or at the least lessen AF progression, ultimately allowing for murine discoveries to translate into practical clinical treatments.

7. Computational models of AF

Atrial fibrillation stands as the most frequently diagnosed cardiac arrhythmia, ensnaring millions globally [1, 2]. The mystique surrounding AF is not merely a product of its prevalence, but stems from a wide variety of causes and mechanisms that drive it. These mechanisms, sprawling across scales from minute molecular interactions to overarching organ dynamics, necessitate an arsenal of sophisticated tools for comprehension. Herein enters the computational model, a digital crucible wherein AF's enigmatic dance can be dissected, offering researchers a panoramic view of its initiation, maintenance, and progression. Insights gleaned from these models not only further the scientific discourse, but also funnel directly into clinical interventions, bridging the chasm between theory and therapeutic application.

Modeling atrial electrical activity and AF, at the theoretical level, involves simulating the spread of an electrical impulse (atrial cell action potential) through a network of connected cells. Most AF models incorporate detailed biophysical properties of membrane protein kinetics, such as ionic channels, pumps, and exchangers. The mathematical foundation of these models is largely built on the formalism developed by Hodgkin and Huxley [101]. In computational AF research, cells are typically arranged in a regular 2- or 3-dimensional network, or in a volumetric model that reflects the geometry and structure of the atria.

7.1 Computational electrophysiological cell models

Early atrial action potential models focused on single cell electrophysiology based on biophysical properties of ion channels, pumps and exchangers [102–104]. These models were used to examine implications of electrical remodeling on potential therapeutic approaches to AF medical management [105]. In more recent computational studies, cellular action potential models have been integrated into structurally realistic cell-coupled models incorporating cardiomechanics [106], regional heterogeneity [107], muscle fiber orientation [108], and patient-specific individualization [109, 110] to develop novel approaches for understanding AF mechanisms and treatment [20, 111].

Peering into the cellular theater of AF, these models render the molecular intricacies of ion movements - the symphony of influxes and effluxes through channels, pumps, and exchangers. As with any scientific tool, the magnifying lens on these models has sharpened over time, adapting to the influx of newer data, particularly human-centric. Not all models are cast in the same mold. While some models sketch the broad contours of AF, others zoom in on the mutations birthed by chronic AF, or explore regions of scientific inquiry that are not readily amenable to in vivo examination, such as effects of fibrillatory substrate size and acetylcholine conditions on rotor maintenance [112].

7.2 Computational models of AF-induced structural remodeling

AF, the ever-evolving maelstrom, often triggers a series of structural shifts in the heart, with fibrosis taking center stage. This scarring of the atrial tissue forms the bedrock of AF's resilience. Computational models, sensing the gravity of fibrosis, have delved deep, by either painting it as non-conductive barricades or by tweaking conduction attributes. The revelations from these models are striking. They spotlight fibrosis as both the anchor for reentrant circuits and the architect of conduction barriers—with either role amplifying AF's stronghold. While lab-based experimental endeavors often grapple with the challenge of segregating the multifaceted roles of fibrosis, computational models allow for explicit investigation of cause and effect. High-definition imagery of atrial fibrosis has infused these models with a granular understanding, empowering them to traverse the fibrotic landscape with unmatched precision and predictive power [113–115].

8. Conclusions

Large and small animal models as well as computational approaches serve as invaluable tools in advancing our understanding of atrial fibrillation. Animal models offer biological context and empirical data, while computational models provide a flexible platform for hypothesis testing and data analysis. The synergistic application of these two methods allows for a more comprehensive understanding of AF. As technology and methodologies evolve, the combined use of these experimental and theoretical approaches will become increasingly crucial for developing effective therapies and achieving a holistic understanding of atrial fibrillation.

Conflict of interest

The authors declare no conflict of interest.

Author details

Rafael J. Ramirez*, Samuel J. Bergman and Jamal A. Masri
Division of Pediatric Cardiac Surgery, Johns Hopkins University School of Medicine, Baltimore, MD, USA

*Address all correspondence to: rjramirez@jhu.edu

References

[1] Benjamin EJ, Wolf PA, D'Agostino RB, Silbershatz H, Kannel WB, Levy D. Impact of atrial fibrillation on the risk of death: The Framingham heart study. Circulation. 1998;**98**(10):946-952

[2] Benjamin EJ, Muntner P, Alonso A, Bittencourt MS, Callaway CW, Carson AP, et al. Heart disease and stroke Statistics-2019 update: A report from the American Heart Association. Circulation. 2019;**139**(10):e56-e528

[3] Lloyd-Jones DM, Wang TJ, Leip EP, Larson MG, Levy D, Vasan RS, et al. Lifetime risk for development of atrial fibrillation: The Framingham heart study. Circulation. 2004;**110**(9):1042-1046

[4] Mou L, Norby FL, Chen LY, O'Neal WT, Lewis TT, Loehr LR, et al. Lifetime risk of atrial fibrillation by race and socioeconomic status: ARIC study (atherosclerosis risk in communities). Circulation. Arrhythmia and Electrophysiology. 2018;**11**(7):e006350

[5] Go AS, Hylek EM, Phillips KA, Chang Y, Henault LE, Selby JV, et al. Prevalence of diagnosed atrial fibrillation in adults: National implications for rhythm management and stroke prevention: The anticoagulation and risk factors in atrial fibrillation (ATRIA) study. Journal of the American Medical Association. 2001;**285**(18):2370-2375

[6] Miyasaka Y, Barnes ME, Gersh BJ, Cha SS, Bailey KR, Abhayaratna WP, et al. Secular trends in incidence of atrial fibrillation in Olmsted County, Minnesota, 1980 to 2000, and implications on the projections for future prevalence. Circulation. 2006;**114**(2):119-125

[7] Di Carlo A, Bellino L, Consoli D, Mori F, Zaninelli A, Baldereschi M, et al. Prevalence of atrial fibrillation in the Italian elderly population and projections from 2020 to 2060 for Italy and the European Union: The FAI project. Europace. 2019;**21**(10):1468-1475

[8] Krijthe BP, Kunst A, Benjamin EJ, Lip GY, Franco OH, Hofman A, et al. Projections on the number of individuals with atrial fibrillation in the European Union, from 2000 to 2060. European Heart Journal. 2013;**34**(35):2746-2751

[9] Chiang CE, Wang KL, Lip GY. Stroke prevention in atrial fibrillation: An Asian perspective. Thrombosis and Haemostasis. 2014;**111**(5):789-797

[10] Tse HF, Wang YJ, Ahmed Ai-Abdullah M, Pizarro-Borromeo AB, Chiang CE, Krittayaphong R, et al. Stroke prevention in atrial fibrillation—an Asian stroke perspective. Heart Rhythm. 2013;**10**(7):1082-1088

[11] Sagris M, Vardas EP, Theofilis P, Antonopoulos AS, Oikonomou E, Tousoulis D. Atrial fibrillation: Pathogenesis, predisposing factors, and genetics. International Journal of Molecular Sciences. 2021;**23**(1):6

[12] Lee S, Khrestian C, Laurita D, Juzbasich D, Wallick D, Waldo A. Validation of a new species for studying postoperative atrial fibrillation: Swine sterile pericarditis model. Pacing and Clinical Electrophysiology. 2023;**46**(8):1003-1009

[13] Tselentakis EV, Woodford E, Chandy J, Gaudette GR, Saltman AE. Inflammation effects on the electrical properties of atrial tissue and inducibility of postoperative atrial fibrillation. The Journal of Surgical Research. 2006;**135**(1):68-75

[14] Kumagai K, Khrestian C, Waldo AL. Simultaneous multisite mapping studies during induced atrial fibrillation in the sterile pericarditis model. Insights into the mechanism of its maintenance. Circulation. 1997;**95**(2):511-521

[15] Chang CJ, Li SJ, Chen YC, Huang SY, Chen SA, Chen YJ. Histone deacetylase inhibition attenuates atrial arrhythmogenesis in sterile pericarditis. Translational Research. 2018;**200**:54-64

[16] Kumagai K, Nakashima H, Urata H, Gondo N, Arakawa K, Saku K. Effects of angiotensin II type 1 receptor antagonist on electrical and structural remodeling in atrial fibrillation. Journal of the American College of Cardiology. 2003;**41**(12):2197-2204

[17] Nattel S, Harada M. Atrial remodeling and atrial fibrillation: Recent advances and translational perspectives. Journal of the American College of Cardiology. 2014;**63**(22):2335-2345

[18] Martins RP, Kaur K, Hwang E, Ramirez RJ, Willis BC, Filgueiras-Rama D, et al. Dominant frequency increase rate predicts transition from paroxysmal to long-term persistent atrial fibrillation. Circulation. 2014;**129**(14):1472-1482

[19] Salvador-Montanes O, Ramirez RJ, Takemoto Y, Ennis SR, Garcia-Iglesias D, Wang S, et al. Panoramic endocardial optical mapping demonstrates serial rotors acceleration and increasing complexity of activity during onset of cholinergic atrial fibrillation. Journal of the American Heart Association. 2021;**10**(22):e022300

[20] Ramirez RJ, Takemoto Y, Martins RP, Filgueiras-Rama D, Ennis SR, Mironov S, et al. Mechanisms by which Ranolazine terminates paroxysmal but not persistent atrial fibrillation. Circulation. Arrhythmia and Electrophysiology. 2019;**12**(10):e005557

[21] Kumagai K, Uno K, Khrestian C, Waldo AL. Single site radiofrequency catheter ablation of atrial fibrillation: Studies guided by simultaneous multisite mapping in the canine sterile pericarditis model. Journal of the American College of Cardiology. 2000;**36**(3):917-923

[22] Creswell LL, Schuessler RB, Rosenbloom M, Cox JL. Hazards of postoperative atrial arrhythmias. The Annals of Thoracic Surgery. 1993;**56**(3):539-549

[23] Goldstein RN, Ryu K, Khrestian C, van Wagoner DR, Waldo AL. Prednisone prevents inducible atrial flutter in the canine sterile pericarditis model. Journal of Cardiovascular Electrophysiology. 2008;**19**(1):74-81

[24] Matsuo K, Uno K, Khrestian CM, Waldo AL. Conduction left-to-right and right-to-left across the crista terminalis. American Journal of Physiology. Heart and Circulatory Physiology. 2001;**280**(4):H1683-H1691

[25] Ortiz J, Niwano S, Abe H, Rudy Y, Johnson NJ, Waldo AL. Mapping the conversion of atrial flutter to atrial fibrillation and atrial fibrillation to atrial flutter. Insights into mechanisms. Circulation Research. 1994;**74**(5):882-894

[26] Uno K, Kumagai K, Khrestian CM, Waldo AL. New insights regarding the atrial flutter reentrant circuit: Studies in the canine sterile pericarditis model. Circulation. 1999;**100**(12):1354-1360

[27] Ishii Y, Schuessler RB, Gaynor SL, Yamada K, Fu AS, Boineau JP, et al. Inflammation of atrium after cardiac surgery is associated with inhomogeneity of atrial conduction

and atrial fibrillation. Circulation. 2005;**111**(22):2881-2888

[28] Burstein B, Nattel S. Atrial fibrosis: Mechanisms and clinical relevance in atrial fibrillation. Journal of the American College of Cardiology. 2008;**51**(8):802-809

[29] Kochiadakis GE, Skalidis EI, Kalebubas MD, Igoumenidis NE, Chrysostomakis SI, Kanoupakis EM, et al. Effect of acute atrial fibrillation on phasic coronary blood flow pattern and flow reserve in humans. European Heart Journal. 2002;**23**(9):734-741

[30] Mariscalco G, Engstrom KG. Postoperative atrial fibrillation is associated with late mortality after coronary surgery, but not after valvular surgery. The Annals of Thoracic Surgery. 2009;**88**(6):1871-1876

[31] Polanczyk CA, Goldman L, Marcantonio ER, Orav EJ, Lee TH. Supraventricular arrhythmia in patients having noncardiac surgery: Clinical correlates and effect on length of stay. Annals of Internal Medicine. 1998;**129**(4):279-285

[32] Heintz KM, Hollenberg SM. Perioperative cardiac issues: Postoperative arrhythmias. The Surgical Clinics of North America. 2005;**85**(6):1103-1114, viii

[33] Gaudino M, Di Franco A, Rong LQ, Piccini J, Mack M. Postoperative atrial fibrillation: From mechanisms to treatment. European Heart Journal. 2023;**44**(12):1020-1039

[34] Fareh S, Benardeau A, Nattel S. Differential efficacy of L- and T-type calcium channel blockers in preventing tachycardia-induced atrial remodeling in dogs. Cardiovascular Research. 2001;**49**(4):762-770

[35] Fareh S, Benardeau A, Thibault B, Nattel S. The T-type Ca(2+) channel blocker mibefradil prevents the development of a substrate for atrial fibrillation by tachycardia-induced atrial remodeling in dogs. Circulation. 1999;**100**(21):2191-2197

[36] Fareh S, Villemaire C, Nattel S. Importance of refractoriness heterogeneity in the enhanced vulnerability to atrial fibrillation induction caused by tachycardia-induced atrial electrical remodeling. Circulation. 1998;**98**(20):2202-2209

[37] Gaspo R, Bosch RF, Bou-Abboud E, Nattel S. Tachycardia-induced changes in Na+ current in a chronic dog model of atrial fibrillation. Circulation Research. 1997;**81**(6):1045-1052

[38] Gaspo R, Bosch RF, Talajic M, Nattel S. Functional mechanisms underlying tachycardia-induced sustained atrial fibrillation in a chronic dog model. Circulation. 1997;**96**(11):4027-4035

[39] Cha TJ, Ehrlich JR, Chartier D, Qi XY, Xiao L, Nattel S. Kir3-based inward rectifier potassium current: Potential role in atrial tachycardia remodeling effects on atrial repolarization and arrhythmias. Circulation. 2006;**113**(14):1730-1737

[40] Cha TJ, Ehrlich JR, Zhang L, Chartier D, Leung TK, Nattel S. Atrial tachycardia remodeling of pulmonary vein cardiomyocytes: Comparison with left atrium and potential relation to arrhythmogenesis. Circulation. 2005;**111**(6):728-735

[41] Cha TJ, Ehrlich JR, Zhang L, Nattel S. Atrial ionic remodeling induced by atrial tachycardia in the presence of congestive heart failure. Circulation. 2004;**110**(12):1520-1526

[42] Morillo CA, Klein GJ, Jones DL, Guiraudon CM. Chronic rapid atrial pacing. Structural, functional, and electrophysiological characteristics of a new model of sustained atrial fibrillation. Circulation. 1995;**91**(5):1588-1595

[43] Li D, Fareh S, Leung TK, Nattel S. Promotion of atrial fibrillation by heart failure in dogs: Atrial remodeling of a different sort. Circulation. 1999;**100**(1):87-95

[44] Jung SW, Sun W, Griffiths LG, Kittleson MD. Atrial fibrillation as a prognostic indicator in medium to large-sized dogs with myxomatous mitral valvular degeneration and congestive heart failure. Journal of Veterinary Internal Medicine. 2016;**30**(1):51-57

[45] Keene BW, Atkins CE, Bonagura JD, Fox PR, Haggstrom J, Fuentes VL, et al. ACVIM consensus guidelines for the diagnosis and treatment of myxomatous mitral valve disease in dogs. Journal of Veterinary Internal Medicine. 2019;**33**(3):1127-1140

[46] Ehrlich JR, Cha TJ, Zhang L, Chartier D, Melnyk P, Hohnloser SH, et al. Cellular electrophysiology of canine pulmonary vein cardiomyocytes: Action potential and ionic current properties. The Journal of Physiology. 2003;**551** (Pt 3):801-813

[47] Ehrlich JR, Cha TJ, Zhang L, Chartier D, Villeneuve L, Hebert TE, et al. Characterization of a hyperpolarization-activated time-dependent potassium current in canine cardiomyocytes from pulmonary vein myocardial sleeves and left atrium. The Journal of Physiology. 2004;**557** (Pt 2):583-597

[48] Verheule S, Wilson EE, Arora R, Engle SK, Scott LR, Olgin JE. Tissue structure and connexin expression of canine pulmonary veins. Cardiovascular Research. 2002;**55**(4):727-738

[49] Dosdall DJ, Ranjan R, Higuchi K, Kholmovski E, Angel N, Li L, et al. Chronic atrial fibrillation causes left ventricular dysfunction in dogs but not goats: Experience with dogs, goats, and pigs. American Journal of Physiology. Heart and Circulatory Physiology. 2013;**305**(5):H725-H731

[50] Chen PS, Chen LS, Fishbein MC, Lin SF, Nattel S. Role of the autonomic nervous system in atrial fibrillation: Pathophysiology and therapy. Circulation Research. 2014;**114**(9):1500-1515

[51] Goldberger AL, Pavelec RS. Vagally-mediated atrial fibrillation in dogs: Conversion with bretylium tosylate. International Journal of Cardiology. 1986;**13**(1):47-55

[52] Sharifov OF, Fedorov VV, Beloshapko GG, Glukhov AV, Yushmanova AV, Rosenshtraukh LV. Roles of adrenergic and cholinergic stimulation in spontaneous atrial fibrillation in dogs. Journal of the American College of Cardiology. 2004;**43**(3):483-490

[53] Olgin JE, Sih HJ, Hanish S, Jayachandran JV, Wu J, Zheng QH, et al. Heterogeneous atrial denervation creates substrate for sustained atrial fibrillation. Circulation. 1998;**98**(23):2608-2614

[54] Schuttler D, Bapat A, Kaab S, Lee K, Tomsits P, Clauss S, et al. Animal models of atrial fibrillation. Circulation Research. 2020;**127**(1):91-110

[55] Burstein B, Comtois P, Michael G, Nishida K, Villeneuve L, Yeh YH, et al. Changes in connexin expression and the atrial fibrillation substrate in congestive heart failure. Circulation Research. 2009;**105**(12):1213-1222

[56] Molina CE, Abu-Taha IH, Wang Q, Rosello-Diez E, Kamler M, Nattel S, et al. Profibrotic, electrical, and calcium-handling remodeling of the atria in heart failure patients with and without atrial fibrillation. Frontiers in Physiology. 2018;**9**:1383

[57] Clauss S, Bleyer C, Schuttler D, Tomsits P, Renner S, Klymiuk N, et al. Animal models of arrhythmia: Classic electrophysiology to genetically modified large animals. Nature Reviews. Cardiology. 2019;**16**(8):457-475

[58] Wijffels MC, Dorland R, Allessie MA. Pharmacologic cardioversion of chronic atrial fibrillation in the goat by class IA, IC, and III drugs: A comparison between hydroquinidine, cibenzoline, flecainide, and d-sotalol. Journal of Cardiovascular Electrophysiology. 1999;**10**(2):178-193

[59] Wijffels MC, Dorland R, Mast F, Allessie MA. Widening of the excitable gap during pharmacological cardioversion of atrial fibrillation in the goat: Effects of cibenzoline, hydroquinidine, flecainide, and d-sotalol. Circulation. 2000;**102**(2):260-267

[60] Wijffels MC, Kirchhof CJ, Dorland R, Allessie MA. Atrial fibrillation begets atrial fibrillation. A study in awake chronically instrumented goats. Circulation. 1995;**92**(7):1954-1968

[61] Wijffels MC, Kirchhof CJ, Dorland R, Power J, Allessie MA. Electrical remodeling due to atrial fibrillation in chronically instrumented conscious goats: Roles of neurohumoral changes, ischemia, atrial stretch, and high rate of electrical activation. Circulation. 1997;**96**(10):3710-3720

[62] Mandapati R, Skanes A, Chen J, Berenfeld O, Jalife J. Stable microreentrant sources as a mechanism of atrial fibrillation in the isolated sheep heart. Circulation. 2000;**101**(2):194-199

[63] Kalifa J, Jalife J, Zaitsev AV, Bagwe S, Warren M, Moreno J, et al. Intra-atrial pressure increases rate and organization of waves emanating from the superior pulmonary veins during atrial fibrillation. Circulation. 2003;**108**(6):668-671

[64] Kalifa J, Tanaka K, Zaitsev AV, Warren M, Vaidyanathan R, Auerbach D, et al. Mechanisms of wave fractionation at boundaries of high-frequency excitation in the posterior left atrium of the isolated sheep heart during atrial fibrillation. Circulation. 2006;**113**(5):626-633

[65] Chen J, Mandapati R, Berenfeld O, Skanes AC, Gray RA, Jalife J. Dynamics of wavelets and their role in atrial fibrillation in the isolated sheep heart. Cardiovascular Research. 2000;**48**(2):220-232

[66] Alvarez-Franco A, Rouco R, Ramirez RJ, Guerrero-Serna G, Tiana M, Cogliati S, et al. Transcriptome and proteome mapping in the sheep atria reveal molecular featurets of atrial fibrillation progression. Cardiovascular Research. 2021;**117**(7):1760-1775

[67] Takemoto Y, Ramirez RJ, Kaur K, Salvador-Montanes O, Ponce-Balbuena D, Ramos-Mondragon R, et al. Eplerenone reduces atrial fibrillation burden without preventing atrial electrical remodeling. Journal of the American College of Cardiology. 2017;**70**(23):2893-2905

[68] Takemoto Y, Ramirez RJ, Yokokawa M, Kaur K, Ponce-Balbuena D, Sinno MC, et al. Galectin-3 regulates atrial fibrillation remodeling and predicts catheter ablation outcomes.

JACC: Basic to Translational Science. 2016;**1**(3):143-154

[69] Takemoto Y, Slough DP, Meinke G, Katnik C, Graziano ZA, Chidipi B, et al. Structural basis for the antiarrhythmic blockade of a potassium channel with a small molecule. The FASEB Journal. 2018;**32**(4):1778-1793

[70] Lenaerts I, Bito V, Heinzel FR, Driesen RB, Holemans P, D'Hooge J, et al. Ultrastructural and functional remodeling of the coupling between Ca^{2+} influx and sarcoplasmic reticulum Ca2+ release in right atrial myocytes from experimental persistent atrial fibrillation. Circulation Research. 2009;**105**(9):876-885

[71] Garrey WE. The nature of fibrillatory contraction of the heart: Its relation to tissue mass and form. American Journal of Physiology. 1914;**33**:397-414

[72] Byrd GD, Prasad SM, Ripplinger CM, Cassilly TR, Schuessler RB, Boineau JP, et al. Importance of geometry and refractory period in sustaining atrial fibrillation: Testing the critical mass hypothesis. Circulation. 2005;**112**(9 Suppl):I7-I13

[73] Nishida K, Michael G, Dobrev D, Nattel S. Animal models for atrial fibrillation: Clinical insights and scientific opportunities. Europace. 2010;**12**(2):160-172

[74] Sugiyama A, Takahara A, Honsho S, Nakamura Y, Hashimoto K. A simple in vivo atrial fibrillation model of rat induced by transesophageal atrial burst pacing. Journal of Pharmacological Sciences. 2005;**98**(3):315-318

[75] Murphy MB, Kim K, Kannankeril PJ, Subati T, Van Amburg JC, Barnett JV, et al. Optimizing transesophageal atrial pacing in mice to detect atrial fibrillation. American Journal of Physiology. Heart and Circulatory Physiology. 2022;**322**(1):H36-H43

[76] Murphy MB, Kim K, Kannankeril PJ, Murray KT. Optimization of transesophageal atrial pacing to assess atrial fibrillation susceptibility in mice. Journal of Visualized Experiments. 2022;**184**:e64168

[77] Halatiu VB, Perian M, Balan AI, Scridon A. Transesophageal atrial burst pacing for atrial fibrillation induction in rats. Journal of Visualized Experiments. 2022;**180**:e63567

[78] Schrickel JW, Bielik H, Yang A, Schimpf R, Shlevkov N, Burkhardt D, et al. Induction of atrial fibrillation in mice by rapid transesophageal atrial pacing. Basic Research in Cardiology. 2002;**97**(6):452-460

[79] Hagendorff A, Schumacher B, Kirchhoff S, Luderitz B, Willecke K. Conduction disturbances and increased atrial vulnerability in Connexin40-deficient mice analyzed by transesophageal stimulation. Circulation. 1999;**99**(11):1508-1515

[80] Ono N, Hayashi H, Kawase A, Lin SF, Li H, Weiss JN, et al. Spontaneous atrial fibrillation initiated by triggered activity near the pulmonary veins in aged rats subjected to glycolytic inhibition. American Journal of Physiology. Heart and Circulatory Physiology. 2007;**292**(1):H639-H648

[81] Haugan K, Lam HR, Knudsen CB, Petersen JS. Atrial fibrillation in rats induced by rapid transesophageal atrial pacing during brief episodes of asphyxia: A new *in vivo* model. Journal of Cardiovascular Pharmacology. 2004;**44**(1):125-135

[82] Boixel C, Fontaine V, Rucker-Martin C, Milliez P, Louedec L,

Michel JB, et al. Fibrosis of the left atria during progression of heart failure is associated with increased matrix metalloproteinases in the rat. Journal of the American College of Cardiology. 2003;**42**(2):336-344

[83] Milliez P, Deangelis N, Rucker-Martin C, Leenhardt A, Vicaut E, Robidel E, et al. Spironolactone reduces fibrosis of dilated atria during heart failure in rats with myocardial infarction. European Heart Journal. 2005;**26**(20):2193-2199

[84] Rucker-Martin C, Milliez P, Tan S, Decrouy X, Recouvreur M, Vranckx R, et al. Chronic hemodynamic overload of the atria is an important factor for gap junction remodeling in human and rat hearts. Cardiovascular Research. 2006;**72**(1):69-79

[85] Choisy SC, Arberry LA, Hancox JC, James AF. Increased susceptibility to atrial tachyarrhythmia in spontaneously hypertensive rat hearts. Hypertension. 2007;**49**(3):498-505

[86] Matsuyama N, Tsutsumi T, Kubota N, Nakajima T, Suzuki H, Takeyama Y. Direct action of an angiotensin II receptor blocker on angiotensin II-induced left atrial conduction delay in spontaneously hypertensive rats. Hypertension Research. 2009;**32**(8):721-726

[87] Ogata T, Ueyama T, Isodono K, Tagawa M, Takehara N, Kawashima T, et al. MURC, a muscle-restricted coiled-coil protein that modulates the rho/ROCK pathway, induces cardiac dysfunction and conduction disturbance. Molecular and Cellular Biology. 2008;**28**(10):3424-3436

[88] Saba S, Janczewski AM, Baker LC, Shusterman V, Gursoy EC, Feldman AM, et al. Atrial contractile dysfunction, fibrosis, and arrhythmias in a mouse model of cardiomyopathy secondary to cardiac-specific overexpression of tumor necrosis factor-alpha. American Journal of Physiology. Heart and Circulatory Physiology. 2005;**289**(4):H1456-H1467

[89] Sah VP, Minamisawa S, Tam SP, Wu TH, Dorn GW 2nd, Ross J Jr, et al. Cardiac-specific overexpression of RhoA results in sinus and atrioventricular nodal dysfunction and contractile failure. The Journal of Clinical Investigation. 1999;**103**(12):1627-1634

[90] Sawaya SE, Rajawat YS, Rami TG, Szalai G, Price RL, Sivasubramanian N, et al. Downregulation of connexin40 and increased prevalence of atrial arrhythmias in transgenic mice with cardiac-restricted overexpression of tumor necrosis factor. American Journal of Physiology. Heart and Circulatory Physiology. 2007;**292**(3):H1561-H1567

[91] Hong CS, Kwon SJ, Cho MC, Kwak YG, Ha KC, Hong B, et al. Overexpression of junctate induces cardiac hypertrophy and arrhythmia via altered calcium handling. Journal of Molecular and Cellular Cardiology. 2008;**44**(4):672-682

[92] Muller FU, Lewin G, Baba HA, Boknik P, Fabritz L, Kirchhefer U, et al. Heart-directed expression of a human cardiac isoform of cAMP-response element modulator in transgenic mice. The Journal of Biological Chemistry. 2005;**280**(8):6906-6914

[93] Adam O, Frost G, Custodis F, Sussman MA, Schafers HJ, Bohm M, et al. Role of Rac1 GTPase activation in atrial fibrillation. Journal of the American College of Cardiology. 2007;**50**(4):359-367

[94] Hirose M, Takeishi Y, Niizeki T, Shimojo H, Nakada T, Kubota I, et al. Diacylglycerol kinase zeta inhibits

G(alpha)q-induced atrial remodeling in transgenic mice. Heart Rhythm. 2009;**6**(1):78-84

[95] Kaese S, Verheule S. Cardiac electrophysiology in mice: A matter of size. Frontiers in Physiology. 2012;**3**:345

[96] Qu Z. Critical mass hypothesis revisited: Role of dynamical wave stability in spontaneous termination of cardiac fibrillation. American Journal of Physiology. Heart and Circulatory Physiology. 2006;**290**(1):H255-H263

[97] Saljic A, Heijman J, Dobrev D. Emerging antiarrhythmic drugs for atrial fibrillation. International Journal of Molecular Sciences. 2022;**23**(8):4096

[98] Si M, Trosclair K, Hamilton KA, Glasscock E. Genetic ablation or pharmacological inhibition of Kv1.1 potassium channel subunits impairs atrial repolarization in mice. American Journal of Physiology. Cell Physiology. 2019;**316**(2):C154-CC61

[99] Wakimoto H, Maguire CT, Kovoor P, Hammer PE, Gehrmann J, Triedman JK, et al. Induction of atrial tachycardia and fibrillation in the mouse heart. Cardiovascular Research. 2001;**50**(3):463-473

[100] Charpentier F, Demolombe S, Escande D. Cardiac channelopathies: From men to mice. Annals of Medicine. 2004;**36**(Suppl 1):28-34

[101] Hodgkin AL, Huxley AF. A quantitative description of membrane current and its application to conduction and excitation in nerve. The Journal of Physiology. 1952;**117**(4):500-544

[102] Courtemanche M, Ramirez RJ, Nattel S. Ionic mechanisms underlying human atrial action potential properties: Insights from a mathematical model. The American Journal of Physiology. 1998;**275**(1):H301-H321

[103] Kneller J, Ramirez RJ, Chartier D, Courtemanche M, Nattel S. Time-dependent transients in an ionically based mathematical model of the canine atrial action potential. American Journal of Physiology. Heart and Circulatory Physiology. 2002;**282**(4):H1437-H1451

[104] Ramirez RJ, Nattel S, Courtemanche M. Mathematical analysis of canine atrial action potentials: Rate, regional factors, and electrical remodeling. American Journal of Physiology. Heart and Circulatory Physiology. 2000;**279**(4):H1767-H1785

[105] Courtemanche M, Ramirez RJ, Nattel S. Ionic targets for drug therapy and atrial fibrillation-induced electrical remodeling: Insights from a mathematical model. Cardiovascular Research. 1999;**42**(2):477-489

[106] Mazhar F, Bartolucci C, Regazzoni F, Paci M, Dede L, Quarteroni A, et al. A detailed mathematical model of the human atrial cardiomyocyte: Integration of electrophysiology and cardiomechanics. The Journal of Physiology. 2023. DOI: 10.1113/JP283974

[107] Calvo CJ, Deo M, Zlochiver S, Millet J, Berenfeld O. Attraction of rotors to the pulmonary veins in paroxysmal atrial fibrillation: A modeling study. Biophysical Journal. 2014;**106**(8):1811-1821

[108] Zhao J, Trew ML, Legrice IJ, Smaill BH, Pullan AJ. A tissue-specific model of reentry in the right atrial appendage. Journal of Cardiovascular Electrophysiology. 2009;**20**(6):675-684

[109] Boyle PM, Ochs AR, Ali RL, Paliwal N, Trayanova NA. Characterizing

the arrhythmogenic substrate in personalized models of atrial fibrillation: Sensitivity to mesh resolution and pacing protocol in AF models. Europace. 2021;**23**(23 Suppl 1):i3-i11

[110] Zahid S, Cochet H, Boyle PM, Schwarz EL, Whyte KN, Vigmond EJ, et al. Patient-derived models link re-entrant driver localization in atrial fibrillation to fibrosis spatial pattern. Cardiovascular Research. 2016;**110**(3):443-454

[111] Pandit SV, Berenfeld O, Anumonwo JM, Zaritski RM, Kneller J, Nattel S, et al. Ionic determinants of functional reentry in a 2-D model of human atrial cells during simulated chronic atrial fibrillation. Biophysical Journal. 2005;**88**(6):3806-3821

[112] Zou R, Kneller J, Leon LJ, Nattel S. Substrate size as a determinant of fibrillatory activity maintenance in a mathematical model of canine atrium. American Journal of Physiology. Heart and Circulatory Physiology. 2005;**289**(3):H1002-H1012

[113] McDowell KS, Vadakkumpadan F, Blake R, Blauer J, Plank G, Macleod RS, et al. Mechanistic inquiry into the role of tissue remodeling in fibrotic lesions in human atrial fibrillation. Biophysical Journal. 2013;**104**(12):2764-2773

[114] Macheret F, Bifulco SF, Scott GD, Kwan KT, Chahine Y, Afroze T, et al. Comparing inducibility of re-entrant arrhythmia in patient-specific computational models to clinical atrial fibrillation phenotypes. JACC: Clinical Electrophysiology. 2023;**9**(10):2149-2162

[115] Roney CH, Sim I, Yu J, Beach M, Mehta A, Alonso Solis-Lemus J, et al. Predicting atrial fibrillation recurrence by combining population data and virtual cohorts of patient-specific left atrial models. Circulation. Arrhythmia and Electrophysiology. 2022;**15**(2):e010253

Section 2

Resynchronization Therapy

Chapter 3

Synchronizing Beats: From Theory to Advances and Insight in Cardiac Resynchronization Therapy

Abdulmohsen Almusaad, Muneera AlTaweel, Abdulrahman Abdullatif Alarfaj, Abdullah Dhawi Al-Otaibi, Mareyah Alshaikh Husain, Rasmah Saad Alharajin, Zainab Albahrani, Yousef Alanazi, Faisal Rabeea Alananzi, Sarah AlMukhaylid and Ahmed Bander Alsalem

Abstract

Cardiac resynchronization therapy (CRT) is an established treatment for select patients with systolic heart failure, left ventricular conduction delay, and dyssynchronous contraction. Landmark trials have shown CRT's benefits on symptoms, exercise capacity, reverse remodeling, hospitalization rates, and mortality. However, limitations exist including sub-optimal patient selection, procedural complexity, high non-responder rates, and device-related adverse effects. This review summarizes the evolution, physiology, clinical trial evidence, patient selection, delivery, and optimization of CRT. Key areas covered include guidelines for CRT use, invasive and noninvasive imaging to improve outcomes, alternative pacing sites to enhance response, and advances in lead technology and implantation techniques. Gaps in current knowledge are highlighted along with future directions for research to refine CRT utilization and improve real-world clinical outcomes. With further studies to address remaining questions, CRT is poised to become an even more effective therapy for heart failure patients with dyssynchronous cardiomyopathy.

Keywords: cardiac resynchronization therapy, CRT clinical trials, QRS duration, left bundle branch area pacing, His pacing, multipoint pacing, scar burden, dyssynchrony, remodeling, CRT responder

1. Introduction

Cardiac resynchronization therapy (CRT) is preferred as a therapeutic approach for individuals presenting with left bundle branch block coupled with symptomatic systolic heart failure, regardless of optimal medical therapy. Guidelines on cardiac resynchronization therapy and cardiac pacing emphasize the importance of CRT in heart failure patients with specific criteria, such as left ventricular ejection fraction (LVEF) $\leq$ 35%, sinus rhythm, and typical left bundle branch block with QRS duration $\geq$150 ms [1]. Advancements in CRT have led to the exploration of alternative pacing sites, the development of newer device-based algorithms, and strategies when traditional CRT is not feasible or effective. Strategies targeting "multi-points" have shown superiority over classic CRT [2]. Additionally, conduction system pacing has arisen as a promising technique [3]. Furthermore, the development of leadless CRT devices has been a significant advancement in this therapy. These devices eliminate the need for traditional leads and are implanted directly into the heart, providing synchronized pacing without the complications associated with lead placement [4]. Successful CRT requires appropriate patient selection, left ventricular lead positioning, and post-implant management. Active research is ongoing to determine how these factors can be optimized to maximize the benefits of CRT [5].

2. Definition of CRT

Cardiac resynchronization therapy or biventricular pacing is a specialized type of pacemaker therapy that provides simultaneous electrical activation of the LV and RV used in patients with LV systolic dysfunction and dyssynchronous ventricular activation [6].

3. Evolution of cardiac resynchronization therapy

3.1 The stepwise evolution of cardiac resynchronization therapy

In 1925, Wiggers conducted canine experiments demonstrating that abnormal electrical activation of the ventricular myocardium led to reduced left ventricular pressure generation (dP/dt) and prolonged isometric contraction. He hypothesized these negative effects of "dyssynchrony" were influenced by the timing of myocardial activation relative to Purkinje fiber excitation. This pioneering work established the mechanistic foundation for cardiac resynchronization [7].

In the 1980s, imaging modalities like radionuclide ventriculography enabled researchers to quantify dyssynchrony's effects on regional cardiac mechanics in humans. Studies by Grines et al. revealed conduction abnormalities like left bundle branch block (LBBB) reduced septal contribution to ventricular ejection and shortened left ventricular filling time, diminishing overall cardiac efficiency (**Figure 1**) [8, 9].

Building on these mechanistic insights, several research groups began exploring whether purposefully pacing different ventricular regions could resynchronize contraction and improve cardiac output:

- Initially described by Befeler et al. in 1978, temporary biventricular pacing was evaluated to treat arrhythmias [10].

- In 1983, Teresa et al. reported improved hemodynamic outcomes in AV block patients with AV sequential pacing [11].

DOI: http://dx.doi.org/10.5772/intechopen.1005299

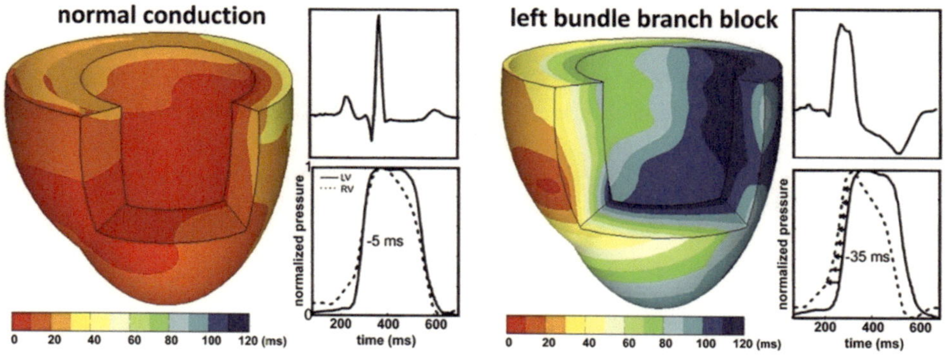

Figure 1.
Typical examples of 3D electrical activation in canine hearts during normal conduction (left) and after creation of left bundle branch block (right). Plotted activation times were derived from ≈110 epicardial and endocardial contact electrodes and referenced to the onset of the Q wave. Electrocardiographic tracings are shown, together with RV and LV pressures signals which are normalized to peak values to reveal timing [8].

- In 1987, Mower patented "biventricular pacing" for heart failure using RV and LV leads [12]. His design included two electrodes: one in the RV and another around the LV free wall, connected in series and programmed to pace after a predetermined AV interval.

- In 1993, Bakker's group tested a dual-chamber pacemaker with a Y adapter on 12 patients with HF and found that biventricular pacing improved functional capacity and left ventricular function [13].

- The pacing system with four chambers, pioneered by Cazeau et al., was observed to increase cardiac output and reduce pulmonary capillary pressure [14].

- Leclercq and team, in 1995, showed that CRT pacing (CRT-P) was more effective than AAI pacing for increasing the cardiac index and reducing pulmonary capillary wedge pressure, demonstrating the benefits of CRT in managing HF [15].

- Auricchio and colleagues found that varying the AV delay for individual patients could optimize the LV dP/dt max and aortic pulse pressure, indicating that CRT response can vary from patient to patient. This understanding led to a focus on personalizing CRT settings for each patient, taking into account factors like QRS duration and morphology, which are now part of the ongoing discussion about AV optimization in CRT [16].

4. Mechanisms of dyssynchrony

4.1 Dyssynchrony and remodeling

Dyssynchrony refers to timing differences in electrical or mechanical activation in the ventricles. It is caused by factors like right ventricular pacing and left bundle branch block (LBBB) [17]. Mechanical dyssynchrony causes inefficient contraction, increasing wall stress over time. This can lead to maladaptive remodeling like hypertrophy and fibrosis [18]. Molecular changes can also impair function in non-dyssynchronous regions [19]. Remodeling causes left ventricular dilation, reduced systolic/diastolic performance, and heart failure symptoms [19].

Chronic RV pacing ≥20–40% or LBBB can induce cardiomyopathy in some patients due to dyssynchrony-mediated remodeling [20]. Measuring mechanical dyssynchrony is important for:

- Detailed assessment beyond electrical dyssynchrony
- Understanding myocyte contraction
- Predicting cardiac resynchronization therapy (CRT) response
- Clinical decision-making in heart failure patients

The mechanisms involved in LBBB dyssynchrony include:

- Delayed LV relaxation and altered diastolic filling [17, 20]
- RV filling precedes LV filling [17]
- Altered LV intracavitary flow patterns [21]
- Impact on global myocardial wall stress during diastole

5. Physiology of biventricular pacing

5.1 Enhanced cardiac physiology through biventricular pacing

Following the implantation of a biventricular pacemaker, cardiac resynchronization therapy (CRT) greatly diminishes cardiac mechanical dyssynchrony, leading to immediate and long-term improvements in heart function and structure. As a result of synchronized ventricular contractions, cardiac output increases immediately. As time progresses, CRT fosters a process of reverse remodeling, evidenced by a reduced left ventricular (LV) size and enhanced LV function (**Figure 2**). These changes are akin to those produced by well-established medications for treating heart failure [22, 23]. These changes are associated with decreased heart failure symptoms and mortality rates (**Figure 3**) [24].

Additionally, CRT can reduce mitral valve dilatation, lessening mitral regurgitation in heart failure patients [25]. On a cellular level, CRT enhances calcium-induced sarcomere contraction and increases beta-adrenergic receptor density, which improves heart muscle contractility and responsiveness [26]. It also boosts energy metabolism by upregulating mitochondrial enzyme activity [27]. However, these benefits are contingent on continued CRT, as discontinuation leads to the loss of therapeutic gains.

6. Major clinical trials

6.1 The core clinical trials

The MUSTIC and PATH-HF studies evaluated the safety and efficacy of CRT in 2001. MUSTIC randomized 67 HF patients to receive CRT for 3 months or no

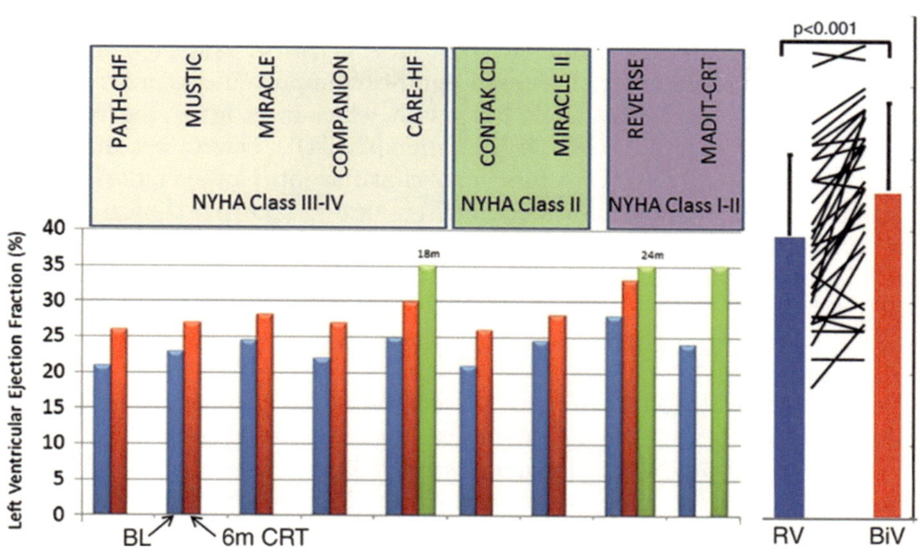

Figure 2.
Change in left ventricular ejection fraction after cardiac resynchronization therapy (CRT) in patients with different functional heart failure classes. Compared with before CRT (blue bars), left ventricular ejection fraction increased significantly in all studies after 3–6 months (red bars) and even more during longer follow-up (green bars). The larger bars on the right indicate data from a study comparing right ventricular (RV) and biventricular (BiV) pacing in pacemaker-dependent patients with mild HF symptoms. The lines indicate the individual response [22].

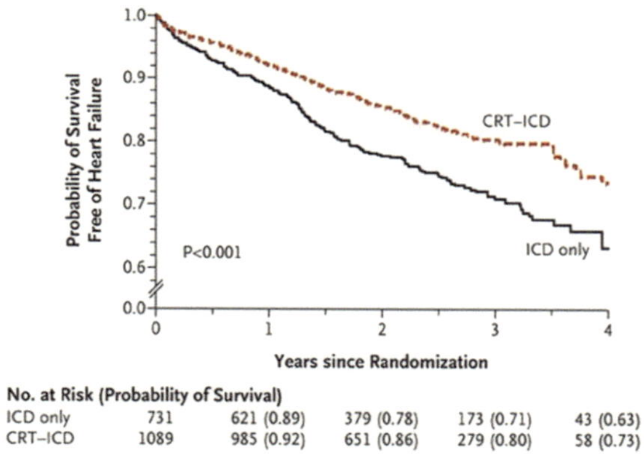

Figure 3.
Kaplan-Meier estimates of the probability of survival free of heart failure. There was a significant difference in the estimate of survival free of heart failure between the group that received cardiac-resynchronization therapy plus an implantable cardioverter-defibrillator (CRT-ICD) and the group that received an ICD only (unadjusted p < 0.001 by the log-rank test) [24].

CRT, showing improvements in walking distance, quality of life, and peak oxygen uptake (VO2) [28]. PATH-HF demonstrated enhanced walking distance and peak VO2 after 12 months of biventricular pacing, along with evidence of left ventricular reverse remodeling [29]. The MIRACLE study, a double-blind trial, randomized 453 HF patients to receive CRT-P or no pacing, observing improvements across various metrics, including left ventricular reverse remodeling, at the 6-month mark [24].

Throughout the 2000s, clinical trials highlighted the advantages of therapy with implantable cardioverter defibrillator (ICD) in patients with impaired left ventricular function. Primary prevention trials showed significant improvements in survival rates with ICDs [30]. The MIRACLE-ICD research, which investigated the impact of supplementing ICD with CRT (CRT-Defibrillation [CRT-D]), determined that CRT-D enhances life quality and the NYHA functional classification. However, the investigation did not extend to walking distance, but it indicated a positive clinical effect without any safety concerns [31]. As the first trial to compare CRT-P and CRT-D with optimal pharmacological therapy (OPT), the COMPANION trial found that CRT-P and CRT-D showed a 20% reduction in mortality or hospitalization, but CRT-D showed the lowest total mortality, demonstrating the benefit of combining CRT and ICD (**Figure 4**) [32, 33].

According to the CARE-HF study, CRT-P reduced cardiovascular hospitalizations, mortality, and quality of life among patients with left ventricular ejection fraction (LVEF) and mitral regurgitation who underwent OPT with or without CRT-P [28]. Despite the therapeutic advantages, the response to CRT varies, with a non-responder rate of 20–40% [34]. Significant clinical trials have refined the understanding and application of CRT. REVERSE (Resynchronization reverses Remodeling in Systolic left ventricular dysfunction) found that CRT induced reverse remodeling in patients with mild heart failure symptoms and left ventricular dysfunction, suggesting benefits from early intervention [35]. MADIT-CRT (Multicenter Automatic Defibrillator Implantation Trial-Cardiac Resynchronization Therapy) demonstrated that CRT reduced hospitalizations due to heart failure in patients with a wide QRS complex and mild symptoms. It emphasized the preventive potential of CRT in halting the progression of heart failure [24].

RAFT (Resynchronization for Ambulatory Heart Failure Trial) included patients with more severe symptoms (NYHA class II–III) and showed a significant mortality reduction for those receiving CRT, confirming the life-saving impact of the therapy in a population with advanced heart failure (**Figure 5**) [36]. Recent trials have also advised against CRT use in patients with narrow QRS complexes and mechanical dyssynchrony, as these patients did not benefit and may even experience harm [23, 37].

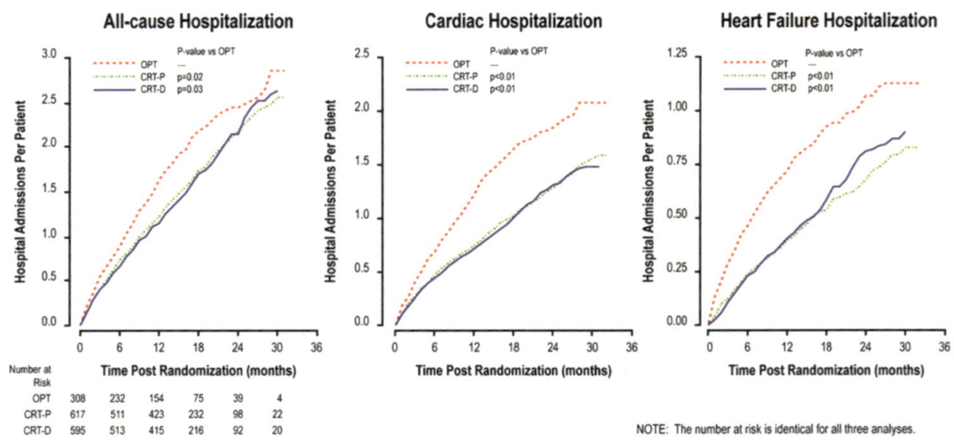

Figure 4.
Hospital admission rate per patient is shown by treatment arm [32].

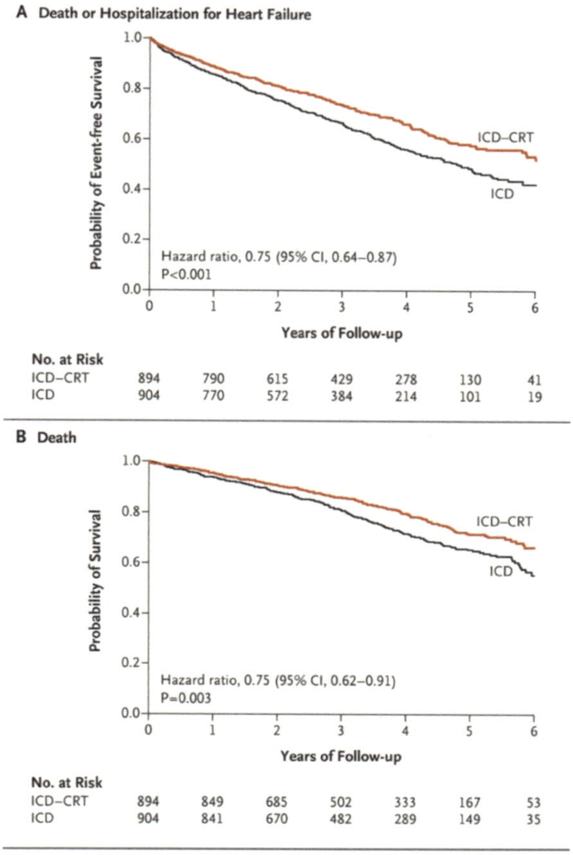

Figure 5.
Kaplan-Meier estimates of death or hospitalization for heart failure (composite primary outcome) and death from any cause. Panel A shows the probability of the primary outcome among patients who were receiving optimal medical therapy along with cardiac-resynchronization therapy (CRT) plus an implantable cardioverter-defibrillator (ICD), as compared with those receiving an ICD alone. The probability of event-free survival at 5 years was 0.576 in the ICD-CRT group and 0.487 in the ICD group. Panel B shows the probability of death from any cause in each group, with a probability of survival at 5 years of 0.714 in the ICD-CRT group and 0.654 in the ICD group [36].

7. Special considerations

7.1 Atrial fibrillation and cardiac resynchronization therapy

A large proportion of trial participants with atrial fibrillation (AF) or heart failure (HF) are excluded from cardiac resynchronization therapy (CRT) trials [38, 39]. A meta-analysis comparing 1164 AF patients with a total of 797 patients with sinus rhythm revealed that AF patients exhibited greater enhancements in ejection fraction. However, AF patients experienced lesser improvements in functional outcomes compared to those in sinus rhythm. Remarkably, in both groups, there was no apparent difference in mortality rates [40].

- CRT devices are programmed to pace only when the heart rate is below a certain threshold, a feature that may present challenges in individuals with atrial fibrillation (AF) characterized by rapid ventricular response. This limitation has the potential to diminish the efficacy of pacing interventions in such patients.

- To ensure CRT delivers maximum benefit, it is essential to control the rate of ventricular contraction by managing AV nodal conduction (**Figure 6**) [41].
- AV nodal conduction can be slowed using medications like beta-blockers, calcium channel blockers, or digoxin.
- In cases where medication is insufficient, catheter ablation of the AV node can induce complete AV block, allowing the CRT device to pace the heart 100% of the time [42].

7.2 Pacing indications and heart failure (HF) risk in bradycardia

The risk of heart failure (HF) is higher for patients with bradycardia who require pacing, regardless of their systolic function status. Conventional pacing typically involves placing a ventricular lead at the right ventricular apex (RVA). However, this can cause left bundle branch block (LBBB) and negatively affect the left ventricular (LV) remodeling and function [43]. To mitigate the risk of HF in these patients, new pacing strategies have been introduced:

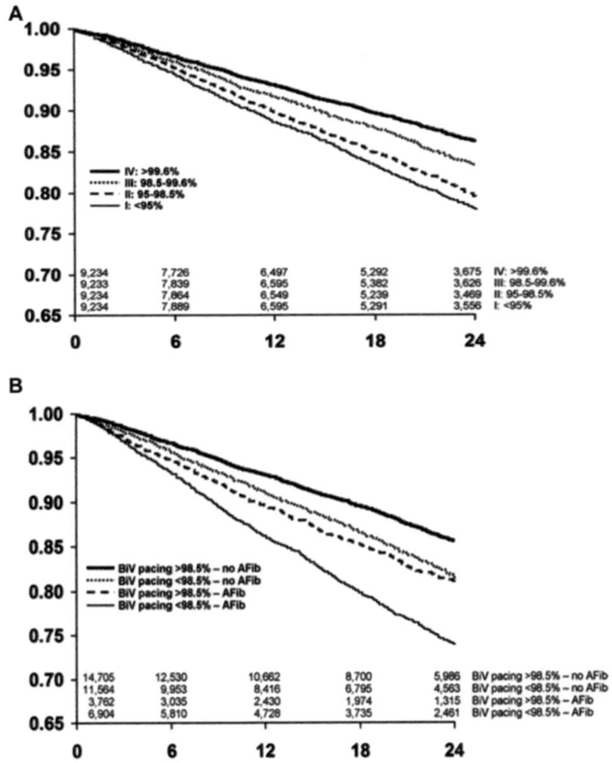

Figure 6.
Survival decreases with reducing biventricular (BiV) pacing in an observational analysis of 36,935 patients with cardiac resynchronization therapy defibrillators. (A) Survival analysis by biventricular pacing percentage. (B) Survival analysis by biventricular pacing percentage and by the presence of significant atrial fibrillation (AFib), defined as average daily burden 0.5% [41].

- Minimizing right ventricular pacing: Specific pacing algorithms can reduce the amount of RVA pacing [44].

- Alternative pacing sites: Septal pacing is considered an option to prevent the dyssynchrony associated with RVA pacing [45].

- Biventricular pacing (CRT): Biventricular pacing is another alternative, and studies have shown its benefits. In the PAVE study, CRT showed superiority over RVA pacing in maintaining ejection fraction (EF) and exercise capacity over 6 months [29]. The APAF study also demonstrated that CRT significantly reduced death from HF, hospitalization due to HF, or worsening HF compared to RVA pacing [46].

- BLOCK HF trial: This trial indicated that CRT is more effective than RV pacing in patients with an LVEF ≤50% and who are expected to pace frequently, reducing mortality, HF-related urgent care visits, and LV dysfunction (**Figure** 7) [47].

- In the PACE study, biventricular pacing was shown to prevent adverse LV remodeling and decreased EF at both 12 and 24 months in patients with normal systolic function. However, the long-term significance of these results is not fully known, and CRTs may carry greater risks of complications [48]. However, the BIOPACE trial compared BiV pacing with RV pacing in 1810 patients with AVB over 5.6 years. The study found no significant difference in death or heart failure hospitalization between the two groups, despite a slight non-significant trend favoring BiV pacing (HR 0.87; p = 0.08). This trend persisted across different LVEF levels but remained statistically insignificant [49].

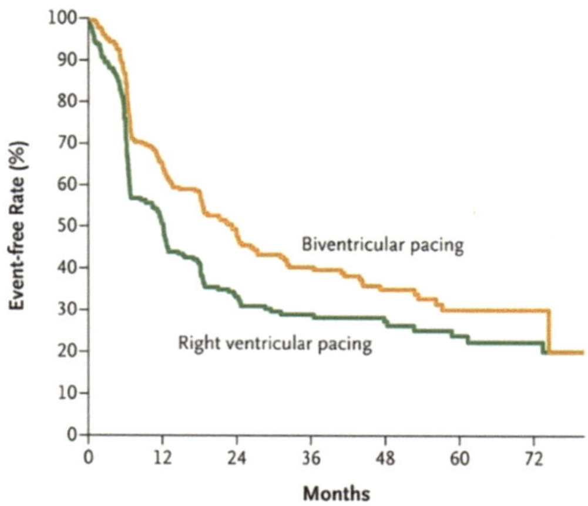

No. at Risk							
Biventricular pacing	349	161	87	62	38	17	3
Right ventricular pacing	342	126	59	39	28	18	10

Figure 7.
Freedom from a primary-outcome event [47].

7.3 Outcomes of CRT-P versus CRT-D

The COMPANION trial in 2004 showed CRT-D reduced all-cause mortality more than CRT-P (36% vs. non-significant trend of 9% reduction), suggesting the superiority of CRT-D [33]. However, the CARE-HF trial in 2005 found CRT-P reduced total mortality compared to medical therapy alone after 29 months of follow-up [29]. A large European registry study of over 1700 patients found CRT-D was superior to CRT-P in reducing mortality over 2 years of follow-up [50]. However, the excess mortality seen with CRT-P was due to non-SCD causes, suggesting a residual risk of SCD was not higher with CRT-P [50]. A nationwide study in England of over 50,000 CRT implantations from 2009 to 2017 reported lower total mortality with CRT-D than CRT-P over a median 2.7 years of follow-up [50].

The risk of SCD is governed by the underlying cardiomyopathy type and timing of CRT implantation. A study analyzing over 15,000 CRT procedures found mortality was lower for non-ischemic cardiomyopathy and when implanted earlier in the disease course [51]. Factors to consider in choosing CRT-D vs. CRT-P include the residual risk of SCD despite CRT (still around 2.7% per year according to recent trials), as well as individual patient characteristics and comorbidities influencing risks of SCD vs. non-SCD death.

8. Patient selection

8.1 Clinical indications and patient selection criteria for CRT

Patients with reduced LVEF and prolonged QRS duration with HF in sinus rhythm should consider CRT; HF in AF patients might also be considered. However, ensuring biventricular capture or return to sinus rhythm is important. Not all HF patients are suitable for CRT—they must meet specific criteria. The main selection criteria are sinus rhythm, LVEF ≤35%, LBBB, QRS ≥150 ms, NYHA class III/IV, on maximal medical therapy. Other criteria that might be considered include AF, LVEF 35–50%, non-LBBB, QRS 130–149 ms, and NYHA class II. CRT is not recommended for QRS <130 ms without an indication of RV pacing (**Tables 1** and **2**) [1, 52, 54].

CRT is strongly recommended	Maybe used
Sinus rhythm	AF
LVEF ≤ 35	LVEF >35 to <50
LBBB QRS morphology	Non-LBBB QRS morphology
QRS complex duration ≥ 150 ms	QRS duration of 130–149 ms
NYHA functional class III or IV	NYHA Class II
Ischemic or nonischemic cardiomyopathy	
Maximal pharmacological therapy for heart failure	
Not recommended: QRS duration < 130 ms without an indication for RV pacing.	

Table 1.
Patient selection for cardiac resynchronization therapy implantation [52].

DOI: http://dx.doi.org/10.5772/intechopen.1005299

	Best candidate	Worst candidate
QRS duration	>150 ms	<120 ms
QRS morphology	LBBB	Nin-LBBB
Scar and dyssynchrony	(−)	(+)
Etiology	CAD (−)	CAD (+)
Gender	Female	Male
Atrial fibrillation	(−)	(+)
CKD	(−)	(+)

CAD, coronary artery disease; CKD, chronic kidney disease; CRT, cardiac resynchronization therapy; LBBB, left bundle branch block.

Table 2.
Patient selection for cardiac resynchronization therapy implantation [53].

8.2 Current guidelines for CRT

The 2021 ESC/EHRA guidelines and 2022 ACC/AHA/HFSA guidelines strongly recommend CRT for symptomatic HF patients in sinus rhythm with LVEF ≤35%, QRS ≥150 ms, and LBBB. The ESC guidelines emphasize CRT for patients requiring RV pacing, while the ACC/AHA/HFSA guidelines assign this a Class IIa recommendation (**Tables 3** and **4**) [52, 55]. For non-LBBB with QRS >150 ms or LBBB with QRS 120–149 ms, CRT should be considered. The ACC/AHA/HFSA guidelines do not recommend CRT for QRS <120 ms, while the ESC guidelines use a cutoff of <130 ms [55].

COR	Recommendations
	LBB QRS morphology
1	CRT is recommended for symptomatic patients with HF in SR with LVEF ≤35%, QRS duration ≥150 ms, and LBBB QRS morphology despite OMT, in order to improve symptoms and reduce morbidity and mortality.
2A	CRT should be considered for symptomatic patients with HF in SR with LVEF ≤35%, QRS duration 130,149 ms, and LBBB QRS morphology despite OMT, in order to improve symptoms and reduce morbidity and mortality.
	Non-LBBB QRS morphology
2A	CRT should be considered for symptomatic patients with HF in SR with LVEF ≤35%, QRS duration ≥150 ms, and non-LBBB QRS morphology despite OMT, in order to improve symptoms.
2B	CRT should be considered for symptomatic patients with HF in SR with LVEF ≤35%, QRS duration 130,149 ms, and non-LBBB QRS morphology despite OMT, in order to improve symptoms and reduce morbidity and mortality.
	QRS duration
3	CRT is not indicated in patients with HF and QRS duration <130 ms without an indication for RV pacing.
	In patients with HF with permanent AF who are candidates for CRT:
2A	CRT should be considered for patients with HF and LVEF ≤35% in NYHA III or IV despite OMT if they are in AF and have intrinsic QRS ≥130 ms, provided a strategy to ensure biventricular capture is in place, in order to improve symptoms and reduce morbidity and mortality.
2A	AVJ ablation should be added in the case of incomplete biventricular pacing (<90–95%) due to conducted AF.

COR	Recommendations
	In patients with symptomatic AF and uncontrolled heart rate are candidates for AVJ ablation (irrespective QRS duration).
1	CRT is recommended in patients with HFrEF.
2A	CRT rather than standard RV pacing should be considered in patients with HFmrEF.
2A	RV pacing should be considered in patients with HFpEF.
2B	CRT may be considered in patients with HFpEF.
2A	Patients who have received a conventional pacemaker or an ICD who subsequently develop symptomatic HF with LVEF ≤35% despite OMT, and who have a significant proportion of PV pacing, should be considered for upgrade to CRT.
	Recommendation for patients with heart failure and atrioventricular block
1	CRT rather than RC pacing is recommended for patients with HFrEF (<40%) regardless of NYHA class who have an indication for ventricular pacing and high-degree AVB in order to reduce morbidity. This includes patients with AF.
	Recommendations for using His bundle pacing
2A	CRT candidates in whom coronary sinus lead implantation is unsuccessful, HBP should be considered as a treatment option along with other techniques such as surgical epicardial lead.
2A	HBP with ventricular backup lead may be considered in patients whom a "pace-and-ablate" strategy for rapidly conducted superventricular arrhythmia is indicated, particularly when the intrinsic QRS is narrow first up.

CLASS (STRENGTH) OF RECOMMENDATION	
CLASS 1 (STRONG)	**Benefit > > > Risk**
Suggested phrases for writing recommendations:	
• Is recommended	
• Is indicated/useful/effective/beneficial	
• Should be performed/administered/other	
• Comparative-Effectiveness Phrases†:	
○ Treatment/strategy A is recommended/indicated in preference to treatment B	
○ Treatment A should be chosen over treatment B	
CLASS 2a (MODERATE)	**Benefit > > Risk**
Suggested phrases for writing recommendations:	
• Is reasonable	
• Can be useful/effective/beneficial	
• Comparative-Effectiveness Phrases†:	
○ Treatment/strategy A is probably recommended/indicated in preference to treatment B	
○ It is reasonable to choose treatment A over treatment B	
CLASS 2b (WEAK)	**Benefit ≥ Risk**
Suggested phrases for writing recommendations:	
• May/might be reasonable	
• May/might be considered	
• Usefulness/effectiveness is unknown/unclear/uncertain or not well-established	

CLASS 3: No Benefit (MODERATE)	
(Generally, LOE A or B use only)	**Benefit = Risk**
Suggested phrases for writing recommendations:	
• Is not recommended	
• Is not indicated/useful/effective/beneficial	
• Should not be performed/administered/other	
Class 3: Harm (STRONG)	**Risk > Benefit**
Suggested phrases for writing recommendations:	
• Potentially harmful	
• Causes harm	
• Associated with excess morbidity/mortality	
• Should not be performed/administered/other	

Table 3.
Recommendation of 2021 ESC guidelines on cardiac pacing and CRT [52].

COR	Recommendations
1	For patients who have LVEF <35% sinus rhythm, left bundle branch block (LBBB) with a QRS duration ≥150 ms, and NYHA class II, III, or ambulatory IV symptoms on GDMT, CRT is indicated to reduce total mortality, reduce hospitalizations, and improve symptoms and QOL. For patients who have LVEF ≤35%, sinus rhythm, LBBB with a QRS duration of ≥150 ms, and NYHA class II, and III, or ambulatory IV symptoms on GDMT, CRT implantation provides high economic value.
2A	For patients who have LVEF ≤35%, sinus rhythm, a non-LBBB pattern with a QRS duration ≥150 ms, and NYHA class II, III, or ambulatory class IV symptoms on GDMT, CRT can be useful to reduce total mortality, reduce hospitalizations, and improve symptoms and QOL.
2A	In patients with high-degree or complete heart block and LVEF of 36–50%, CRT is reasonable to reduce total mortality, reduce hospitalizations, and improve symptoms and QOL.
2A	For patients who have LVEF ≤35%, sinus rhythm, LBBB with QRS duration 120–149 ms, and NYHA class II, III, or ambulatory IV symptoms on GDMT, CRT can be useful to reduce total mortality, reduce hospitalizations, and improve symptoms and QOL.
2A	In patients with AF and LVEF ≤35% on GDMT, CRT can be useful to reduce total mortality improve symptoms and QOL, and increase LVEF, if: (a) the patient requires ventricular pacing or otherwise meets CRT criteria (b) atrioventricular nodal ablation or pharmacological rate control will allow near 100% ventricular pacing with CRT.
2A	For patients on GDMT who have LVEF ≤35% and are undergoing placement of a new or replacement device implantation with anticipated requirement for significant (>40%) ventricular pacing, CRT can be useful to reduce total mortality, reduce hospitalizations, and improve symptoms and QOL.
2B	For patients who have LVEF ≤35%, sinus rhythm, a non-LBBB with QRS duration of 120–149 ms, and NYHA class III or ambulatory class IV on GDMT, CRT can be useful to reduce total mortality, reduce hospitalizations, and improve symptoms and QOL.
2B	For patients who have LVEF ≤30%, ischemic cause of HF, sinus rhythm, LBBB with QRS duration ≥150 ms, and NYHA class I symptoms on GDMT, CRT may be considered to reduce hospitalizations and improve symptoms and QOL.
3	In patients with QRS duration <120 ms, CRT is not recommended.
3	For patients with NYHA I or II symptoms and non-LBBB pattern with QRS duration <150 ms, CRT is not recommended.
3	For patients comorbidities or frailty limit survival with good functional capacity to <1 year, ICD and cardiac resynchronization therapy with defibrillation (CRT-D) are not indicated.

CLASS (STRENGTH) OF RECOMMENDATION	
CLASS 1 (STRONG)	**Benefit > > Risk**
Suggested phrases for writing recommendations:	
• Is recommended	
• Is indicated/useful/effective/beneficial	
• Should be performed/administered/other	
• Comparative-Effectiveness Phrases†:	
○ Treatment/strategy A is recommended/indicated in preference to treatment B	
○ Treatment A should be chosen over treatment B	
CLASS 2a (MODERATE)	**Benefit > > Risk**
Suggested phrases for writing recommendations:	
• Is reasonable	
• Can be useful/effective/beneficial	
• Comparative-Effectiveness Phrases†:	
○ Treatment/strategy A is probably recommended/indicated in preference to treatment B	
○ It is reasonable to choose treatment A over treatment B	
CLASS 2b (WEAK)	**Benefit ≥ Risk**
Suggested phrases for writing recommendations:	
• May/might be reasonable	
• May/might be considered	
• Usefulness/effectiveness is unknown/unclear/uncertain or not well-established	
CLASS 3: No Benefit (MODERATE)	
(Generally, LOE A or B use only)	**Benefit = Risk**
Suggested phrases for writing recommendations:	
• Is not recommended	
• Is not indicated/useful/effective/beneficial	
• Should not be performed/administered/other	
Class 3: Harm (STRONG)	**Risk > Benefit**
Suggested phrases for writing recommendations:	
• Potentially harmful	
• Causes harm	
• Associated with excess morbidity/mortality	
• Should not be performed/administered/other	

Table 4.
2022 AHA/ACC/HFSA guidelines for the management of heart failure [55].

8.3 QRS criteria in CRT

The definition of left bundle branch block (LBBB) varies across medical guidelines and studies, affecting how patients are classified and recommended for cardiac resynchronization therapy (CRT). This inconsistency may lead to improper inclusion or exclusion of patients [56, 57]. Some researchers have proposed redefining LBBB criteria by considering gender differences in ventricular wall thickness and requiring septal activation patterns on ECG [57]. Complications also arise in patients with LBBB after myocardial infarction [58]. Studies show that strict ECG criteria, like QS or rS in V1, mid-QRS notching, and absence of Q in lateral leads, are associated with better CRT outcomes (**Tables 5** and **6**) [59].

	Responders (n = 75)	**Non-responders (n = 27)**	**p-Value**
PR interval	162.2 ± 23.0	182.2 ± 32.3	0.02
QRS duration	172.4 ± 21.9	170.7 ± 24.2	n.s.
LBBB morphology	77.3%	66.7%	n.s.
R amplitude in V1	1.1 ± 0.4	1.3 ± 0.5	0.04
S amplitude in V1	14.2 ± 5.9	14.5 ± 6.8	n.s.
R amplitude in V6	6.6 ± 5.0	3.6 ± 2.9	0.01
S amplitude in V6	4.1 ± 3.9	7.3 ± 6.6	0.01
R6/S6	4.6 ± 5.4	1.7 ± 2.5	0.02
(S1 + R6) − (S6 + R1)	15.7 ± 10.8	9.5 ± 8.8	0.02
Paced QRS duration	127.5 ± 26.3	137.0 ± 23.2	0.08

Table 5.
Electrocardiographic variable in responder and non-responder group [59].

Predictors of CRT response	**Predictors of CRT non-response**
True LBBB	
• QRS duration ≥130 ms in women and ≥140 ms in men • Mid-QRS notching and/or slurring in two contiguous leads in V1–2 or I-aVL, V5–V6 • Absence of q waves in the lateral leads • Absence of R wave in V1 (≥1 mm) • 45 ms ≤ between the peak of the R to the nadir of the S wave in V1	
Non-true LBBB and non-LBBB	
• QRS duration ≥150 ms • Mid-QRS notching or/and slurring in one lateral lead • Masquerading bundle branch block • ID in lead V6 > 60 ms • QR-max index >120 ms	• More than two notches on the R wave or the nadir of the S wave. • <32.5 ms to the beginning of the QRS fragmentation from the QRS onset and a longer fractionation duration • Lead one ratio < 12
All QRS morphologies	
• ID in lead I ≥ 110 ms • ID in lead aVL ≥ 130 ms • ID/QRS duration >0.69 in lead I • [ID in lead I-ID in lead V1] >90 ms • [aVLID-aVFID]/QRSd >25% • [V5ID-V1ID]/QRSd >25% • Large R/S in V6 (absence of deep S wave)	• QRS duration <130 ms

Table 6.
Useful electrocardiographic signs to support the prediction of favorable response to cardiac resynchronization therapy [59].

According to trials such as MADIT-CRT and RAFT, patients with left bundle branch block (LBBB) benefit more from CRT than those with right bundle branch block (RBBB) or intraventricular conduction delay (IVCD) [30, 60]. While CRT trials historically used QRS ≥ 150 ms, evidence now supports QRS > 120–130 ms, especially in sicker patients. However, guidelines still advise CRT for QRS ≥ 150 ms or ≥ 130 ms + LBBB based on trials like MADIT-CRT, REVERSE, and RAFT (**Figure 8**) [28, 60, 61]. A meta-analysis shows CRT is effective for QRS ≥ 150 ms but not <150 ms [61]. Clinicians can be optimistic about CRT response for QRS ≥ 150 ms, particularly non-LBBB patients. More data are needed for Class I patients.

8.4 CRT and narrow QRS complex

CRT has undergone assessment for patients exhibiting a QRS duration <120 ms, resulting in different outcomes. While initial investigations conducted at single centers proposed symptomatic improvements in this population subset following CRT, findings from extensive trials have contradicted these findings.

Particularly, the LESSER-EARTH trial (Evaluation of Resynchronization Therapy for Heart Failure) and the EchoCRT (Echocardiography-Guided Cardiac Resynchronization Therapy) study, both multicenter, randomized, controlled trials, failed to indicate a mortality advantage with the incorporation of CRT to an Implantable Cardioverter Defibrillator (ICD) among this patient cohort [62, 63].

In the LESSER-EARTH trial, CRT did not improve clinical outcomes or lead to left ventricular (LV) reverse remodeling. There was even an indication that CRT could potentially be harmful [62, 63]. The EchoCRT trial focused on patients with a QRS duration of 130 ms or less, Left Ventricular Ejection Fraction (LVEF) of 35% or less, and mechanical dyssynchrony. In this investigation, participants underwent implantation of CRT-Defibrillator (CRT-D) devices and were subsequently randomly allocated to

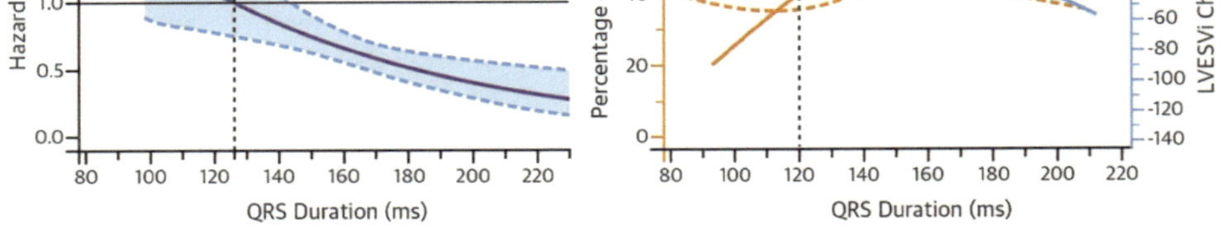

Figure 8.
Central Illustration relation between QRS duration and the response and outcome of cardiac resynchronization therapy. (Left) Taken from a meta-analysis of individual patient data from landmark cardiac resynchronization therapy (CRT) trials showing hazard ratios (y-axis and solid purple line) 95% confidence interval (CI) (blue shading) for effects on total mortality of CRT versus control patients, with QRS duration plotted on the x-axis using spline smoothing. The intersection between the solid purple line and the vertical dashed line at a hazard ratio of 1.0 (no effect) denotes the QRS duration above which there is a high certainty of response. (Right) Data from a subanalysis of the REVERSE study showing the proportion of patients with an improved clinical response (CRT in solid gold line and control in dashed gold line) and the absolute change in left ventricular end-systolic volume index (LVESVi) at 12 months (CRT in solid blue line and control patients in dashed blue line) [59].

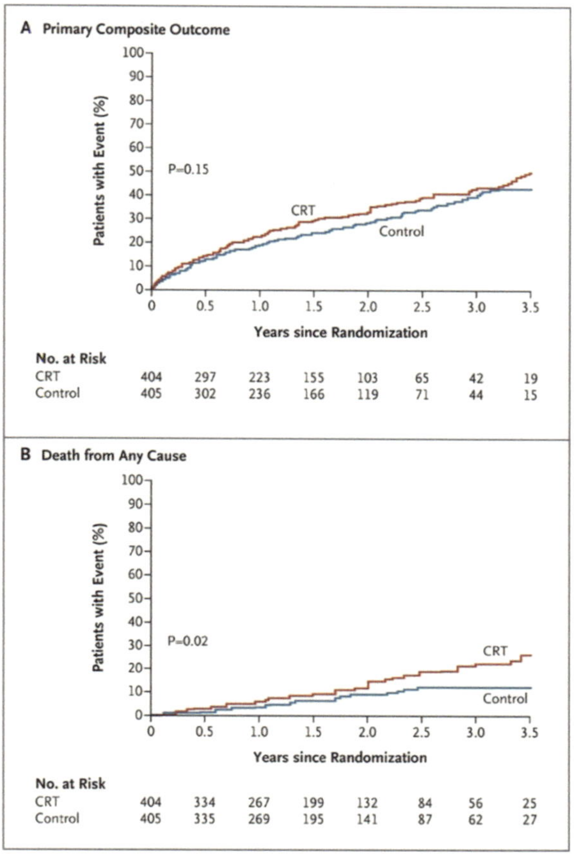

Figure 9.
Echo-CRT trial cardiac-resynchronization therapy in heart failure with a narrow QRS complex Kaplan-Meier estimates for primary-outcome events. Panel A shows the Kaplan-Meier curves for the primary composite outcome of death from any cause or hospitalization for heart failure. Panel B shows the Kaplan-Meier curves for death from any cause [63].

either activate or deactivate the CRT function. The trial was prematurely terminated due to futility, as there was noted to be a rise in mortality rates in patients receiving CRT-D (**Figure 9**) [63]. These findings suggest that extending CRT to patients with shorter QRS durations may not provide the expected benefits and could even be detrimental, challenging the rationale for using CRT in this subset of heart failure patients.

9. Predictors of response

9.1 Non-responders to cardiac resynchronization therapy

Approximately 33% of patients do not show a hemodynamic improvement following the therapy (**Figure 10**). The relevance of measuring individual responses to CRT is questioned, as this is not a common practice in other medical interventions that aim for an average treatment effect, acknowledging that some patients will not benefit regardless [64]. Non-response rates for heart failure drugs like enalapril, bisoprolol, and spironolactone are high, suggesting that lack of response might be influenced by

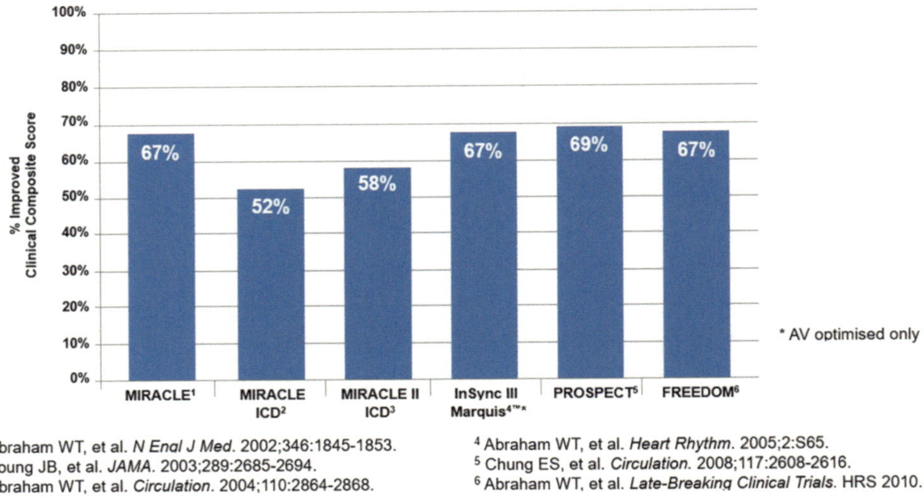

Figure 10.
30% of CRT patients are non-responders.

genetic factors. However, the challenge remains to identify a reliable surrogate marker for prognostic response to CRT. LV reverse remodeling is suggested as one such surrogate because of its predictive value for cardiovascular mortality. Yet, it is not perfect as it does not predict symptomatic improvement and could lead to misclassification of non-responders.

Other potential surrogate markers like peak VO2 and natriuretic peptides have their limitations, with the former weakly predicting mortality and the latter being too variable to be useful in clinical practice. Factors known to reduce the response to CRT include increased scar burden, certain scar locations, extreme mechanical dyssynchrony, and comorbidities like severe right ventricular dysfunction, pulmonary hypertension, renal failure, and valvular disease (**Figure 11**) [65]. However, without studies comparing these factors to control patients on optimal therapy, their impact on CRT effectiveness is not clear. Preventing the deterioration of a patient's condition could be considered a response to CRT, though this effect has not been quantified in research. Gender and the cause of heart failure are noted to influence CRT outcomes, with women and those with nonischemic HF etiology generally experiencing better results from CRT [66].

9.2 Electrocardiographic parameters as predictors of response to CRT

While no single ECG parameter could predict CRT response on its own, yet specific parameters did demonstrate a difference between responders and non-responders. In particular, an increased amplitude of the R wave in lead V6, an elevated R/S ratio in the same lead, and the derived figure (S1 + R6) – (S6 + R1) may suggest a greater likelihood of response in both LBBB and non-LBBB patients [67].

ECG variables: (S1 + R6) – (S6 + R1): This computed variable involves the summation of the S wave in lead V1 and the R wave in lead V6, subtracted from the sum of the S wave in lead V6 and the R wave in lead V1. The significant difference in this variable between responders and non-responders suggests that the spatial and temporal characteristics of ventricular depolarization, as reflected on the ECG, might correlate with the mechanical synchrony achieved through CRT [68].

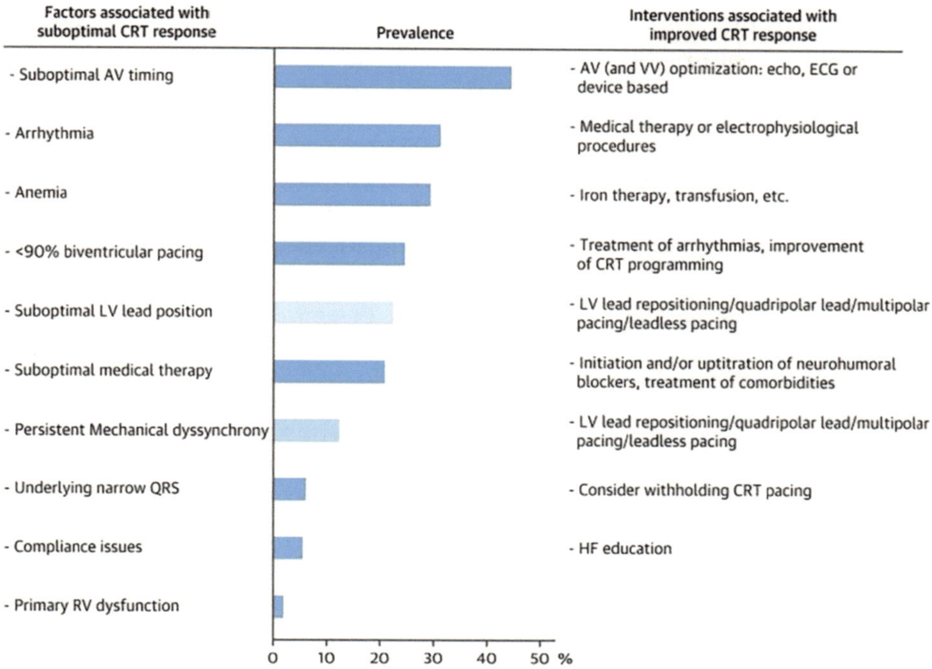

Figure 11.
Factors associated with sub-optimal CRT response [65].

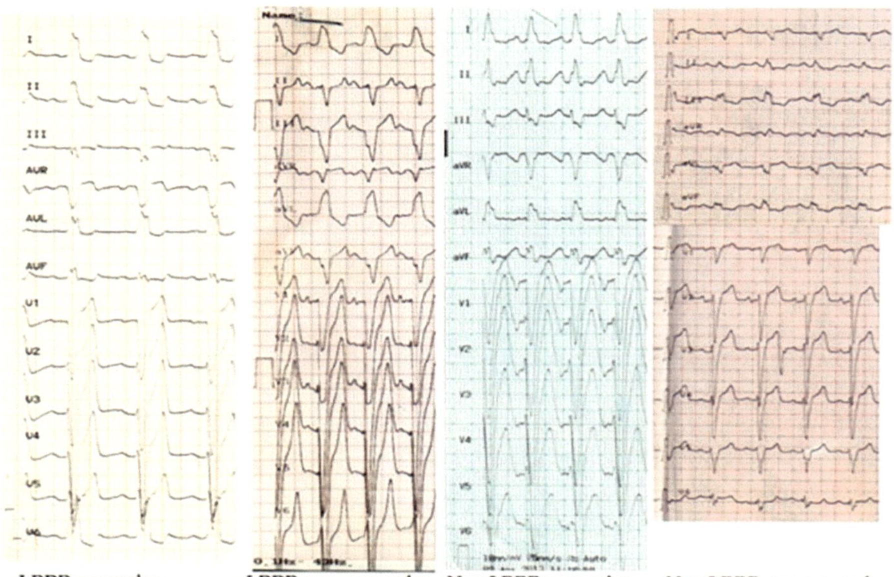

Figure 12.
LBBB responder and non LBBB responder.

R6/S6 ratio: The ratio of the R wave to the S wave amplitude in lead V6 provides an index of the electrical activity in the lateral wall of the left ventricle. A higher R6/S6 ratio in responders may indicate a more favorable left ventricular electrical substrate for CRT [69].

Height of R wave in V6: The R wave amplitude in the V6 lead represents the electrical forces directed toward the lateral wall of the left ventricle. A higher amplitude might correlate with less scarring and better contractile reserve in the lateral wall, which could translate into a better response to CRT [70].

LBBB vs. Non-LBBB Patients: Patients with LBBB typically have a more dyssynchronous contraction pattern, and CRT aims to correct this dyssynchrony. Therefore, parameters that reflect the extent of dyssynchrony in LBBB patients may be more predictive of CRT response in this group compared to non-LBBB patients (**Figure 12**) [67, 71].

9.3 The role of imaging

9.3.1 Imaging for patient selection

9.3.1.1 Echocardiography

- Early investigations indicated that echocardiographic assessments of mechanical dyssynchrony were indicative of the outcome of cardiac resynchronization therapy (CRT) [72]. Nevertheless, recent trials have observed that echocardiographic evaluations of dyssynchrony lacked consistent reliability in predicting CRT response. Clinical recommendations have subsequently shifted away from employing echocardiographic dyssynchrony as a criterion for patient selection for cardiac resynchronization therapy (CRT) [1, 73]

9.3.1.2 Cardiac magnetic resonance (CMR) and dyssynchrony

- CMR, especially myocardial tagging, offers a sophisticated method for assessing myocardial motion [74].

- Despite some measures of dyssynchrony via CMR showing promise in predicting CRT outcomes, they lack external validation.

- Complicating its use in predicting CRT response, mechanical dyssynchrony is influenced by various factors beyond conduction disturbances, including myocardial perfusion, viability, and passive motion [1].

9.3.1.3 Imaging to guide left ventricular (LV) pacing

- While dyssynchrony imaging may not be ideal for selecting patients, it has the potential to optimize LV lead placement [75].

- The TARGET and STARTER trials indicated that echocardiography could help improve CRT outcomes by targeting late-activated myocardial segments [75].

- CT imaging of coronary veins and CMR to avoid pacing in scarred areas are other strategies [1].

- Emerging techniques include electroanatomic and ECG body surface mapping, as well as image fusion and computational modeling to assist in LV lead positioning [76].

9.3.1.4 Scar burden

- A higher scar burden has been associated with a lower response rate to CRT in CMR and nuclear imaging studies [76].
- However, a specific cutoff for scar burden that predicts CRT response has not been established or validated [1].
- The assessment of scar burden and its clinical implications in CRT continues to be a research focus.

10. Optimizing outcomes

10.1 Enhancing CRT outcomes by targeting the LV pacing site

10.1.1 Current CRT implantation technique

- The transvenous technique for CRT, established in 1994, remains standard practice [77].
- A posterolateral LV lead placement with good pacing parameters and no diaphragmatic stimulation is the typical goal [77].
- Studies yield conflicting results; some suggest lead position on the LV free wall is not crucial, while others find non-apical positions more favorable [78].

10.1.2 Variability in patient response

- Even with appropriate fluoroscopic positioning, patient responses to CRT are variable [29]. Fluoroscopic imaging does not account for myocardial factors that affect pacing efficacy [78].

10.1.3 Targeting late-activated segments

- Recent approaches focus on implanting LV leads in segments of the heart that activate late to improve CRT response (**Figure 13**) [79, 80].
- The STARTER trial (Echocardiography-guided left ventricular lead placement for cardiac resynchronization therapy) found this method reduced death or HF hospitalization but achieved only 30% accuracy in targeting late-activated segments (**Figure 14**) [81].
- Scarring was not considered in these results, raising questions about the influence of myocardial scarring on outcomes [50].

10.1.4 Influence of myocardial scarring

- Pacing in scarred myocardium correlates with a poorer response to CRT [82].

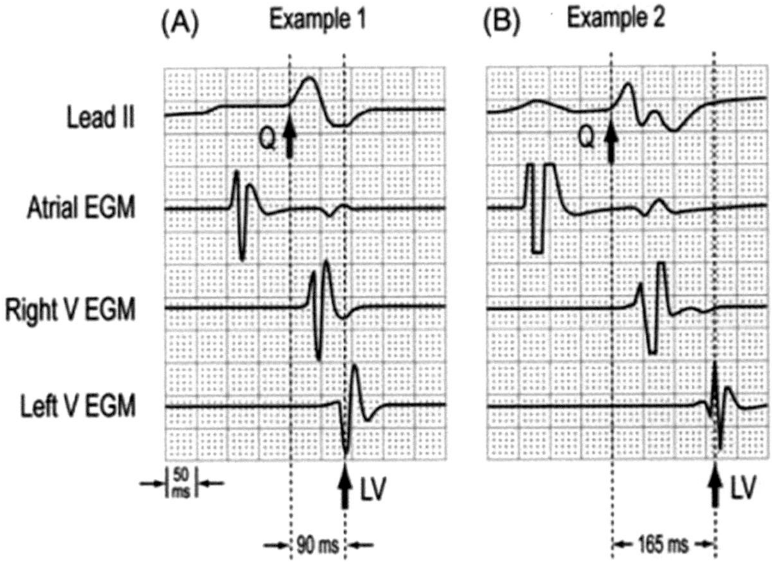

Figure 13.
Examples of QLV measurements. The calipers are aligned with the onset of QRS and peak of the left ventricular electrogram. The QLV was calculated as 90 ms for the patient in (A) and 165 ms for the patient in (B) [79].

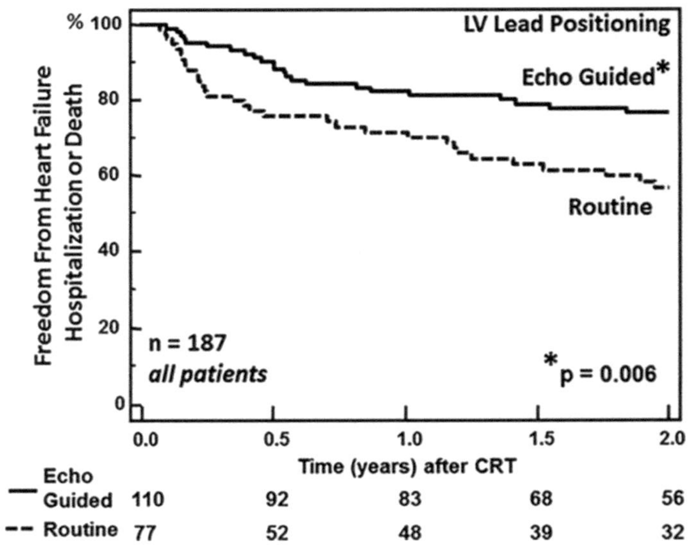

Figure 14.
Kaplan-Meier plots of the results of the primary end point of freedom from heart failure hospitalization or death after cardiac resynchronization therapy (CRT), including all randomized patients with intention-to-treat analysis. Patients randomized to echocardiographic guided left ventricular (LV) lead positioning strategy had a significantly more favorable clinical outcome in comparison to routinely treated patients [81].

- The degree of scarring intensifies the negative impact on CRT efficacy [82].
- CMR-guided pacing to avoid scarred tissue seems beneficial, but further validation is needed [82].

DOI: http://dx.doi.org/10.5772/intechopen.1005299

10.1.5 Enhancing the response by multipolar LV leads

Multipoint pacing (MPP) in cardiac resynchronization therapy (CRT) has revealed improving clinical outcomes and reversing left ventricular (LV) remodeling associated with heart failure [83]. In a randomized, multicenter study conducted in the Middle East, patients implanted with CRT-D devices were randomized to receive either biventricular pacing (BiV) or MPP therapy. According to the study, a higher proportion of MPP patients had a reduction in end-systolic volume (ESV) of 15% or more and improved NYHA functional class than those with BiV (**Figure 15**) [84].

Moreover, a systematic review and meta-analysis comparing multipoint pacing (MPP) to traditional biventricular (BiV) pacing revealed that MPP correlated with a

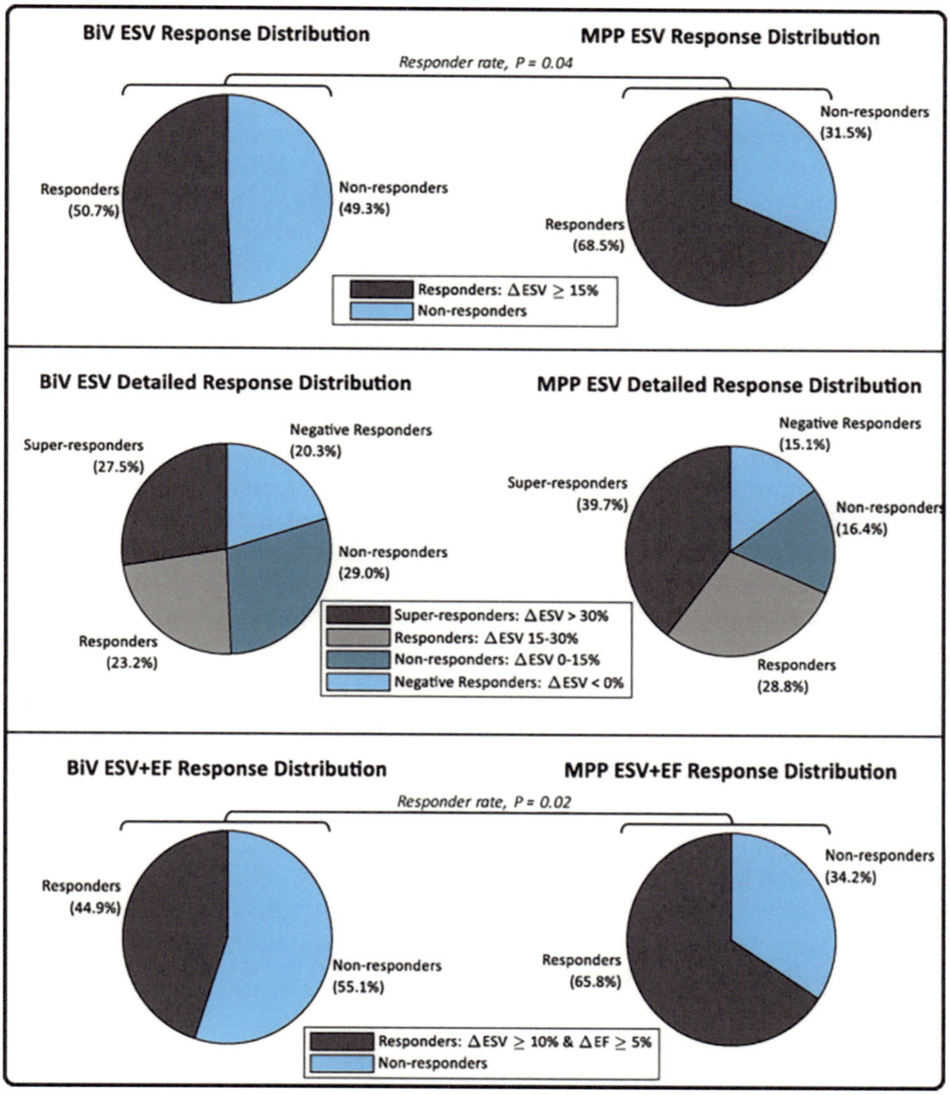

Figure 15.
End-systolic volume (ESV) response distribution (top), detailed ESV response distribution (middle), and end-systolic volume + ejection fraction (ESV + EF) response distribution (bottom) for biventricular (BiV) and multipoint pacing (MPP) patients [84].

heightened occurrence of patients experiencing functional improvement and elevated delta left ventricular (LV) dP/dtmax, suggesting enhanced hemodynamic parameters. Despite no notable variance between MPP and BiV in terms of hospitalization for heart failure, LV end-systolic volume, and all-cause mortality, MPP was associated with significantly lower projected battery longevity. These findings suggest that MPP has the potential to improve functional class and acute hemodynamic parameters in patients with heart failure, yet additional investigation is needed to understand the long-term advantages and optimize programming strategies for MPP [83]. Multipolar LV leads also offer the possibility of avoiding diaphragmatic stimulation and selecting from multiple pacing vectors [76]. This technology might enable specific targeting of viable and late-activated myocardium [76]. Although promising, more evidence is required to confirm whether multipolar leads enhance CRT outcomes [76]. Preference for multipolar leads is increasing, potentially making them the new standard [76].

10.2 Device optimization to enhance CRT response

Device optimization in cardiac therapy is crucial to improve left ventricular (LV) function, which is affected by atrioventricular (AV) delays. While echocardiography has traditionally been employed for identifying optimal AV delays, its time-consuming nature has led to its decline in busy medical settings. Instead, operators often use a trial-and-error approach to find the best device settings, which is not methodologically robust. Furthermore, echocardiographic optimization, despite being a gold standard, has not been proven to enhance outcomes and may be no more effective than using standard device settings [85].

Automatic, device-based AV and VV (ventriculo-ventricular) optimization offer practical benefits over manual methods. However, studies have shown mixed results. The FREEDOM study revealed that the QuickOpt algorithm was less effective than echocardiographic optimization [85]. Similarly, the Smart-AV study found that the Smart-AV algorithm did not result in LV reverse remodeling when compared to standard settings [76]. Adaptive CRT, which uses an algorithm for automatic selection of pacing mode and AV/VV optimization, was shown to be comparable to echocardiographic optimization in the Adaptive CRT study (**Figure 16**) [53, 85]. Nonetheless, it remains uncertain if these benefits are due to the optimization of AV/VV intervals or the pacing mode itself [76].

10.3 Possible solutions for non-responders

10.3.1 Alternative pacing

Lead-based endocardial LV pacing and conduction system pacing like His bundle pacing (HBP) and left bundle branch area pacing (LBBAP) can improve outcomes for non-responders to standard biventricular pacing. HBP activates the physiological conduction system but has limitations like difficult implantation, high pacing thresholds, and early battery depletion [86].

10.3.2 His-bundle pacing

His bundle pacing restores physiological activation of the ventricles. It has shown feasibility and efficacy for managing arrhythmias and heart failure [87–91]. However, it has drawbacks such as challenging implantation, unstable pacing thresholds, the risk of crosstalk, and failure to achieve cardiac resynchronization in some patients.

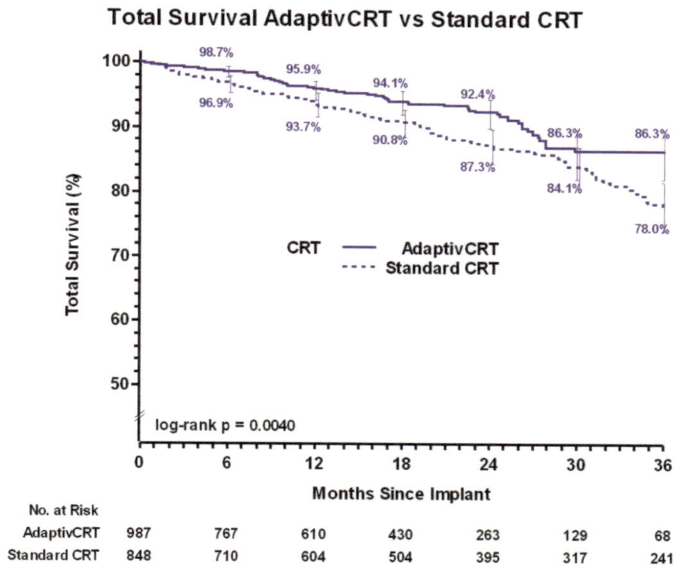

Figure 16.
End-improved survival with dynamic optimization of CRT pacing using adaptive CRT algorithm: analysis of real world patient data [53].

Limitations include prolonged procedures, high thresholds, early battery depletion, and lead dislodgement (**Figure 17**) [92–94].

10.3.3 Left bundle branch area pacing

In the evolving landscape of cardiac resynchronization therapy (CRT), left bundle branch area pacing (LBBAP) has emerged as a promising alternative to traditional

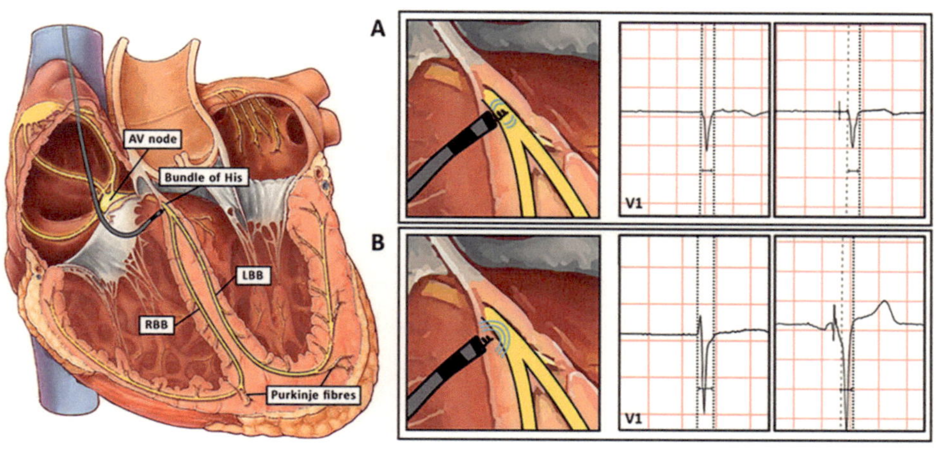

Figure 17.
Forms of His bundle pacing. (A) During selective His bundle (HB) capture, ventricular activation occurs directly over the His-Purkinje system. There is an isoelectric line between the pacing stimulus and the QRS which is identical to the native QRS. (B) In nonselective HB pacing there is fusion capture of HB and adjacent myocardial tissue resulting in the presence of pseudo-delta wave. Although paced QRS duration is slightly increased (by the H-QRS interval), the overall electrical axis of the paced QRS is concordant with the electrical axis of the intrinsic QRS [92].

approaches. While HBP has shown promise in CRT, it is not without its challenges. The presence of potential blockages along the conduction system can hinder the effectiveness of HBP. To overcome these obstacles, researchers have proposed stimulating the conduction system distal to the His bundle, specifically targeting the left bundle branch. This distal approach aims to bypass areas of blockage and achieve a more profound and targeted form of cardiac resynchronization (**Figure 18**).

LBBAP has gained attention as a practical, safe, and promising option in the realm of CRT. Its versatility extends beyond patients who have experienced unsuccessful Biventricular Pacing (BVP)-CRT implantation or are non-responders. LBBAP is also being considered as a primary choice for addressing intraventricular conduction delay [95]. The technique involves pacing either the main trunk of the left bundle branch or its anterior/posterior fascicles, with a preference for the main trunk in cases of the left bundle branch block. In cases lacking conduction abnormalities, especially those with a narrow QRS, left bundle branch area pacing (LBBAP) provides a distinct advantage. Through retrograde activation of the right bundle branch, LBBAP can promptly stimulate the right ventricle with minimal delay. This approach aids in preserving interventricular synchrony and potentially achieving physiological ventricular synchrony. As a result, LBBAP is proving to be a suitable pacing strategy, especially in the context of pure anti-bradycardia pacing without intraventricular conduction abnormalities [96, 97].

Recent studies have shed light on the comparative effectiveness of LBBAP in relation to other pacing strategies. The left bundle branch pacing vs. left ventricular septal pacing vs. Biventricular Pacing for Cardiac Resynchronization Therapy trial demonstrated superior clinical outcomes with LBBAP compared to LVSP and BIVP for CRT patients [53]. Achieving left bundle branch capture appeared to be a crucial factor in the success of LBBAP, while LVSP and BIVP showed no significant differences. This prospective, multicenter study involving 415 patients undergoing CRT further solidified the position of LBBAP as the preferred pacing strategy based on the research findings [98].

Left bundle branch area pacing represents a promising frontier in the field of cardiac resynchronization therapy and is regarded as an excellent choice for BVP-CRT for patients with left ventricular dysfunction and conduction abnormalities. Further research is crucial to affirm the potential significance of these pacing techniques and to deepen our understanding of their similarities and differences [53, 97].

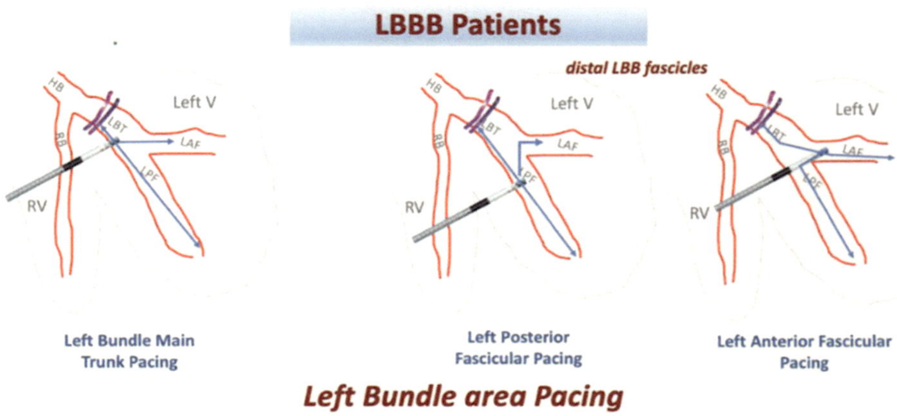

Figure 18.
Left bundle area pacing in left bundle branch block patients targets zones [86].

DOI: http://dx.doi.org/10.5772/intechopen.1005299

10.3.4 Left bundle branch area pacing procedural protocol

The goal of conduction system pacing is to produce a more physiologic ventricular activation sequence that resembles normal ventricular activation during sinus rhythm. This goal can be achieved either by capturing the HIS bundle directly at the base of the interventricular septum (IVS) or by capturing the left bundle, which is located more distally on the IVS. Of the two techniques, left bundle branch area pacing (LBBAP) has emerged as the most attractive of the two techniques given higher sensing amplitude, lower capture threshold and greater degree of stability, and low number of lead revisions [99, 100]. Thus, only LBBAP technique will be discussed in this section.

From its inception, LBBAP has been performed almost exclusively using lumen-less pacing leads (LLL-LBBAP), mainly the SelectSecure 3830 (Medtronic Inc., Minneapolis, USA). Alternatively, standard-stylet-driven pacing leads (SDL-LBBAP) have been reported to be both safe and practical [101]. Although the lead and helix designs differ, the implantation technique is similar for both leads. Both techniques use a delivery sheath to deliver the lead at a more perpendicular angle to the IVS to allow for lead migration into the septum, as indicated in **Figure 19**. In patients presenting with left bundle branch block (LBBB), backup ventricular pacing is highly recommended, given the possibility of transient complete AV block due to mechanical pressure on the HIS bundle.

10.3.4.1 LBBAP implantation steps

10.3.4.1.1 Identification of the initial site of implantation on the septum

The sheath and dilator are advanced to the RV over a guidewire, this is best achieved in right anterior oblique (25-degree) view. Once the delivery system is in the RV, the dilator and wire are withdrawn, and the lead is advanced to the tip of the sheath. The Ideal location for lead fixation is 1–1.5 cm apical to the HIS location in the RV septum. This can be achieved by connecting electronic clips to the lead in a unipolar fashion and sensing HIS bundle depolarization to determine the starting point in the RV. Alternatively, pacing from the lead tip and observing the paced morphology, can help locate the optimal site for lead fixation. The ideal pacing morphology as shown in **Figure 20** includes the following:

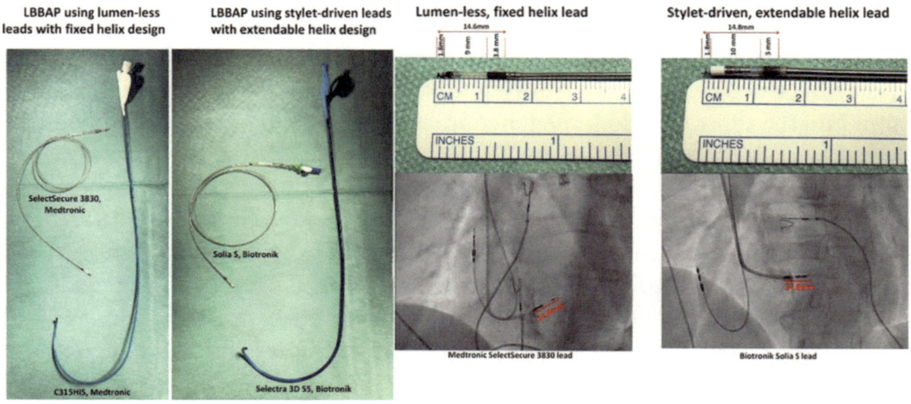

Figure 19.
Lumen-less and style-driven leads used in LBBAP and corresponding delivery sheaths.

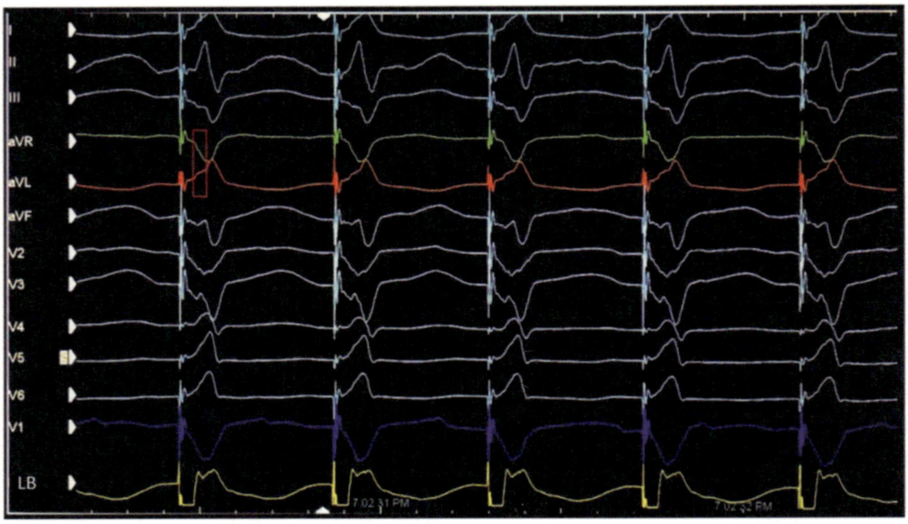

Figure 20.
Target pacing morphology at the RV septum to indicate an adequate site for lead fixation.

- W pattern in V1, with a hump or notch on the later half preferably
- R wave is taller in lead II than III
- aVR and aVL discordance in the first 40 ms

Once an adequate unipolar pacing morphology is observed, contrast injection of the sheath is helpful to assess the apposition of the sheath to the septum, this is usually performed in the lateral anterior oblique view (20–25 degrees). A satisfactory contrast injection should show near perpendicular alignment on the interventricular septum. This location should be stored as a reference to assess lead placement into the septum.

10.3.4.1.2 Lead deployment and advancement into the septum

Lead advancement into the septum requires clockwise rotation of the lead with forward pressure while monitoring lead migration into the septum on fluoroscopy. The lead can be observed to rotate during forward displacement. Approximately 6–8 mm into the septum, lead impedance as well as pacing morphology should be evaluated.

Pacing morphology following initial rotation should be assessed, as the lead migrates into the septum the notch in V1 will start to move later in the QRS, ultimately, the notch will reach the end of the QRS and an R′ will be observed. Although this is usually observed during LBBAP, it is not a universal finding and adequate final locations can only show a notch in V1 in the later half with terminal negative electrical force. Once the lead helix reaches the LV sub-endocardium, a sudden reduction in the QRS duration typically occurs, along with a decrease in the left ventricular activation time (LVAT), indicating successful capture of the LV conduction system. LVAT is defined as the interval from pacing stimulation to the appearance of R waves in leads V4–V6 (**Figure 21A**).

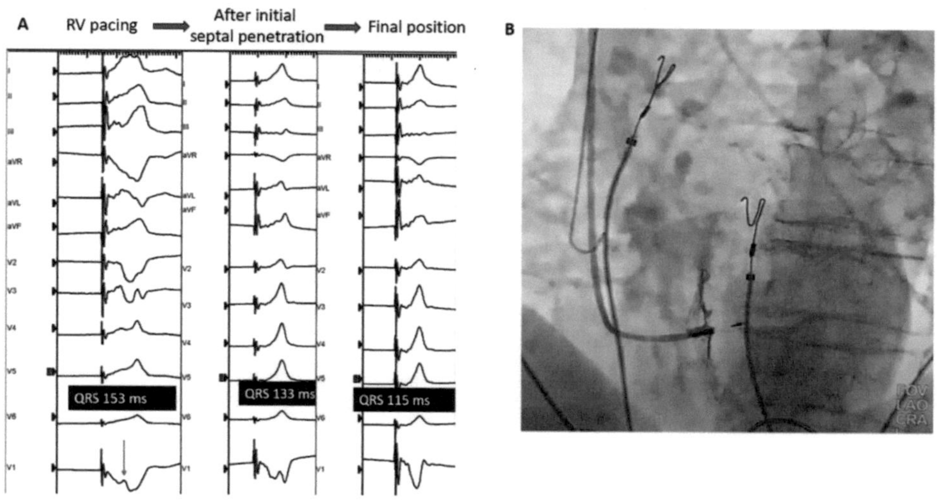

Figure 21.
(A) Progression of unipolar pacing morphology during lead fixation into the ventricular septum. (B) Sheath contrast injection showing extent of septal lead migration.

Initial impedance is expected to be relatively high during penetration. As the lead migrates into the septum, lead impedance will start to gradually decrease, signaling deep penetration into the septum and proximity to the left ventricular endocardium. Generally, unipolar lead impedance should be >500 Ohms. Sheath contrast injection can help determine lead implantation depth into the septum, as well as identify inadvertent septal perforation (**Figure 21B**).

10.3.4.1.3 Determining final lead position

The final lead position should show a pacing morphology that reflects a terminal R′ in V1 and LVAT of less than 90 ms, this usually is accompanied by a narrow QRS of less than 120 ms. When the left ventricular conduction system is captured with the lead helix, a low pacing threshold (<1.5 V/0.5 ms) is usually observed. Observing fixations beats which are premature ventricular depolarizations (VPD) with RBBB morphology with left axis deviation signifies mechanical stimulation of the left posterior fascicle, this finding indicates proximity to LV endocardium, and further migration into the septum should be avoided [102]. Left bundle potentials can be recorded once the lead helix is in proximity to the LV endocardium. Once the final location is reached, bipolar pacing should be performed, and pacing impedance and bipolar capture threshold determined. Following sheath removal, adequate lead slack should be ensured to prevent lead dislodgement or migration, and a 12-lead ECG is recommended to document pacing morphology immediately following implantation (**Figure 22**).

10.3.4.1.4 Septal perforation and septal artery injury

Septal lead perforation into the LV cavity can occur due to excessive lead rotation and migration into the septum. This is indicated by a marked decrease in pacing impedance that corresponds with sudden increase in unipolar capture threshold. Fluoroscopy usually shows deep penetration of the lead from the site of initial

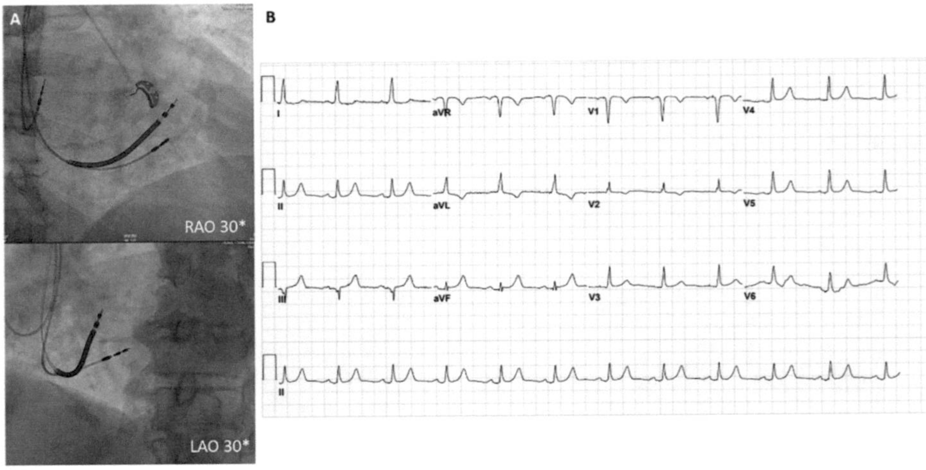

Figure 22.
(A) Final lead location in a patient who underwent CRT-D placement with a left bundle branch area pacing following failed CS cannulation due to lack of acceptable CS branches. (B) ECG showing LBBAP with narrow QRS of 88 ms and LVAT of 72 ms.

implantation. Sheath contrast injection can show contrast escape into the LV cavity. If septal perforation occurs, withdrawal of the lead into the RV is usually possible without major consequences as the lead track into the septum is sealed by septal muscle rebound and rarely leaves residual connection between the right and left ventricle. The lead should be removed from the sheath and examined for any retained muscle tissues as this will hinder lead re-implantation.

Septal perforator artery injury can occur during LBBAP lead implantation, this can be minimized by placing the lead inferiorly and posteriorly on the septum to avoid the large septal branches usually observed in the anterior septum. Contrast injection into the delivery sheath can delineate septal vascular injury [103].

10.3.5 Endocardial left ventricular (LV) pacing

Endocardial pacing seems to produce more efficient resynchronization than epicardial pacing. It allows pacing from a variety of LV sites without restrictions from coronary sinus anatomy [104]. Potential advantages of endocardial LV pacing include optimizing the pacing site to target the latest activation area based on evidence from trials like TARGET, which showed echo-guided targeting had superior response compared to empirical placement [1]. Studies show endocardial pacing accesses fast-conducting tissue or Purkinje fibers for faster LV activation than epicardial pacing and may reduce arrhythmogenic effects by restoring physiological activation/repolarization patterns [105].

Lead-based endocardial LV pacing was used in the ALSYNC trial of 132 patients, which reported 55% had reverse remodeling and 59% symptomatic improvement at 6 months [106]. However, it is limited by thromboembolic risk requiring anticoagulation. The WiSE-CRT leadless system avoids these risks. The SELECT-LV trial of 35 patients showed a high 97.1% procedural success and 84.8% clinical response at 6 months [107]. An international WiSE-CRT registry of 90 patients demonstrated good procedural success at 94.4% and 69.8% clinical response at 6 months **Figures 23** and **24** [98, 104, 108]. Endocardial LV pacing warrants further research into leadless delivery systems as a promising option for CRT non-responders.

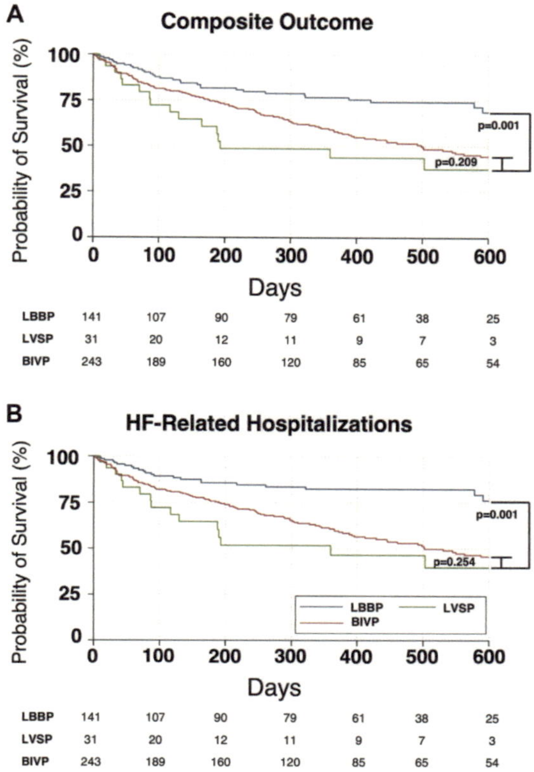

Figure 23.
(A) Primary composite outcome. (B) Heart failure (HF)-related hospitalization. Left bundle branch pacing vs. left ventricular septal pacing vs. biventricular pacing for cardiac resynchronization therapy [98].

11. Procedural techniques

11.1 Pre-implant patient evaluation

Before cardiac resynchronization therapy (CRT) implantation, a comprehensive patient evaluation is crucial. The European Society of Cardiology and the European Heart Rhythm Association have provided guidelines for this process [109]. The assessment should include a detailed medical history, physical examination, vital signs, and laboratory tests to ensure that patients have stable heart failure (HF) while on guideline-directed medical therapy (GDMT) [109].

Echocardiography plays a vital role in measuring left ventricular ejection fraction (LVEF) and assessing cardiac size and function. Additionally, a 12-lead electrocardiogram (ECG) is necessary to evaluate QRS duration and morphology [109]. For patients at high risk of thromboembolism receiving warfarin, maintaining treatment at a lower dose while monitoring the international normalized ratio (INR 2–3) is recommended, with postoperative heparin being discouraged [109].

Prophylactic treatment with antibiotics that target staphylococcal bacteria is recommended [109]. Also, performance of quality life (QOL) functionality assessments to assess the anticipated response to cardiac resynchronization therapy (CRT) is advised [109]. Cardiac magnetic resonance imaging (cMRI) and computed tomography angiography (CTA) can both reflect valuable insights into myocardial viability and venous anatomy, respectively.

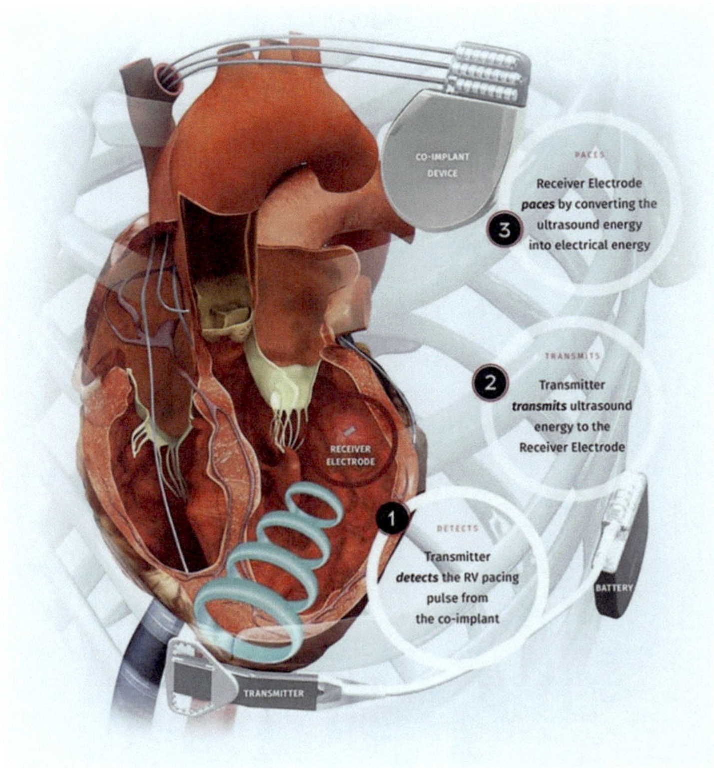

Figure 24.
Endocardial LV pacing—components of the WiSE-CRT system [104].

Identifying and managing atrial fibrillation or frequent premature ventricular contractions (PVCs) that may hinder continuous CRT therapy delivery is essential [109]. For patients with a low to moderate risk of thromboembolism, changing the anticoagulant therapy dose before surgery is recommended to minimize bleeding risk [109]. CRT should be postponed in patients with HF, on inotrope medication, or with unstable ventricular arrhythmias [25]. Patients should not be excluded from cardiac resynchronization therapy based on echocardiographic dyssynchrony assessment [25].

If a patient is decompensated with HF, dependent on inotropes, or has unstable ventricular arrhythmias, CRT should be postponed until the medical condition improves [25]. The assessment of dyssynchrony in the echocardiogram should not be used to rule out patients for CRT [25].

11.2 Perioperative period

Close monitoring post-CRT implantation is essential due to potential changes in urine output and electrolyte balance, which may necessitate modifications to the prescribed drugs [110]. Temporarily withdrawing antiplatelet agents before implantation may decrease bleeding risk [111]. Perioperative antibiotic administration has been shown to significantly reduce infection rates [110].

Despite technological advancements and improved surgical techniques, complications such as LV lead failure, hematomas, dissections, perforations, heart block, lead

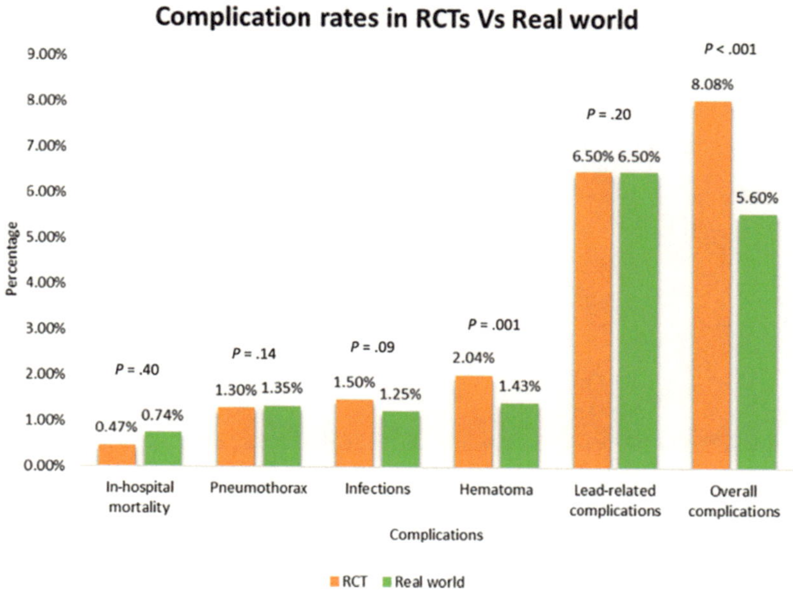

Figure 25.
Rates of reported complications of cardiac resynchronization therapy in randomized controlled trials, registries, and administrative databases [112].

dislodgement, renal failure, and mortality can occur, with overall complication rates ranging from 4% to 28% (**Figure 25**) [110, 113].

11.3 Targeting LV lead placement

Optimal LV lead placement and stability are critical for successful CRT outcomes [110, 114, 115]. Conventional lead implantation involves placing a single LV lead through the coronary sinus (CS) into a suitable vein, with the target vein selected based on anatomical considerations. Fluoroscopic guidance and operator experience are used for optimal site determination (**Figure 26**) [110, 114, 115]. However, this approach has limitations, including subjective assessment and potentially suboptimal positioning.

Research has shown that apically positioned LV leads are associated with poorer clinical outcomes [110]. While the COMPANION and MADIT-CRT trials demonstrated comparable responses between lateral, anterior, or posterior locations, the REVERSE trial patients benefited from lateral positions [110]. Imaging techniques may assist in selecting specific LV pacing sites based on anticipated electromechanical optimization [110].

11.4 Techniques for CRT implantation

Techniques for CRT implantation as recommended by The European Society of Cardiology [109].

11.4.1 Pre-procedural considerations

- Patient assessment and imaging to understand venous anatomy.
- Selection of equipment based on the patient's anatomical requirements.

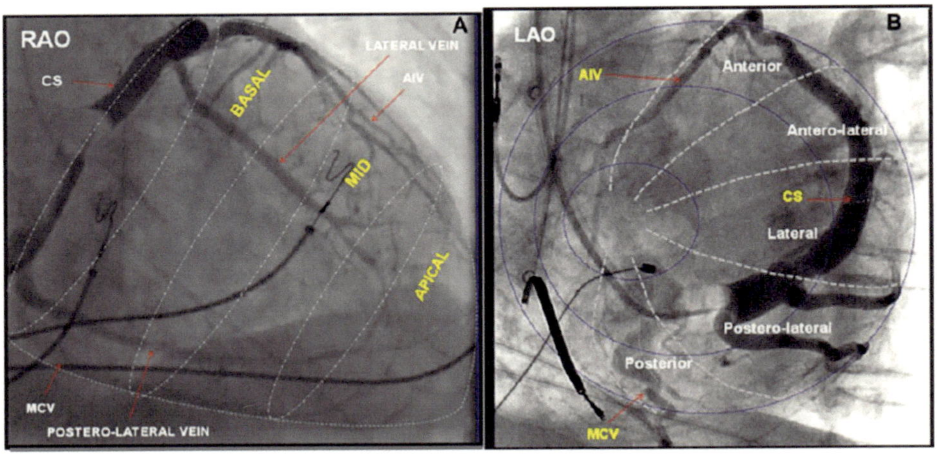

Figure 26.
CS venous tributaries and segments of the left ventricle [116].

11.4.2 Sedation and anesthesia

- Conscious sedation and local anesthesia are the norms.
- General anesthesia for special cases such as pediatric patients or those who cannot be sedated under normal circumstances.

11.4.3 Pacing leads placement sequence

1. *Right ventricular (RV) lead*: Establish baseline pacing.
2. *Left ventricular (LV) lead*: Critical for resynchronization, placed using the sheath in the CS branch.
3. *Right atrial (RA) lead*: Placed last to complete the setup.

11.4.4 LV lead positioning

- Obtaining a detailed phlebogram to visualize the CS anatomy.
- Selecting a target vein based on size, absence of stenosis, and location.
- Aim for proximal to mid-third of the LV to match areas of greatest dyssynchrony.

11.4.5 Branch cannulation techniques

- Customizing approaches to patient-specific anatomy, such as using specialized catheters or leads.
- Maneuvers for difficult angles including inner catheters or leads with special curves.

11.4.6 Lead stability and placement troubles

- Ensuring lead stability with designs meant for aggressive fixation or active fixation mechanisms.
- Stenting as a method to secure a lead position.
- Exploring alternative venous branches or sheath shapes for challenging anatomy.
- Post-implantation assessment including electronic repositioning and chest radiography [112].

11.4.7 Post-procedure management

- Monitoring complications such as diaphragmatic capture or threshold variations.
- Chest X-ray to confirm final lead placement and for future comparisons.

Potential need for reprogramming or repositioning leads electronically in case of issues [109].

11.5 Implantation tips and tricks

Difficult LV lead implantations in CRT can be attributed to various factors such as difficulty accessing the coronary venous system, anatomic variations, scar tissue, phrenic nerve stimulation, and lead instability. By utilizing new technologies, improved tools, and techniques, clinicians can overcome these challenges and improve the success rates of CRT implantations for heart failure patients [112].

Potential Causes of Difficult LV Lead Implantations and Solutions:

Failure to access the coronary venous system: Difficulty in accessing the coronary venous system is a common cause of implant failure. Improved technology, such as specific sheaths with primary and secondary curves, allows better support and cannulation of the coronary sinus (CS). Techniques like withdrawing the sheath with counterclockwise rotation and using contrast dye injections for better visualization can aid in accessing the CS [117].

Anatomic variations in the coronary venous system: Upon successful cannulation of the coronary sinus (CS), and obtaining a venogram, the CS anatomy is recognized. In case of failure, alternative imaging modalities like venous-phase coronary angiography, computed tomography (CT)-guided imaging, fiberoptic endoscopy, or intracardiac echocardiography can be used. Specially shaped sheaths and inner catheters can be used for lead delivery in challenging vessel segments [112].

Extensive scar tissue in the target region: Scar tissue can make lead implantation difficult. Techniques such as careful dissection of the scar tissue, use of guidewires or inner catheters for support, and consideration of alternative lead placement sites can help overcome this challenge [116].

Phrenic nerve stimulation: Phrenic nerve stimulation can occur during LV lead implantation, causing diaphragmatic contraction. Proper lead positioning, pacing adjustments, or using multipolar leads can help avoid or manage phrenic nerve stimulation [118].

LV lead instability: LV lead instability can lead to poor pacing outcomes. Techniques like using fixation screws, atraumatic leads, and active fixation leads can enhance lead stability and reduce the risk of dislodgement [112].

11.6 Delivery of CRT in the real world

Cardiac resynchronization therapy (CRT) has been shown to provide incremental survival benefits to optimal pharmacotherapy (OPT) in patients with advanced heart failure (HF), according to the IMPROVE HF study [119]. Moreover, recent evidence suggests CRT may slow disease progression even in mild HF cases. Despite these benefits, the adoption rate of CRT remains low [50]. HF significantly impacts both survival rates and quality of life, with non-CRT patients experiencing a mortality rate comparable to certain cancers, as indicated by the CARE-HF study. Yet, the treatment of HF with CRT has not reached the same level of comprehensive patient coverage as seen in oncology for those with both advanced and early-stage disease [120]. Additionally, CRT is not without its complications, which must be considered. One of the key barriers to effective CRT delivery is the separation between the fields of HF and electrophysiology. A multidisciplinary approach is crucial, requiring a shift in focus to ensure that patients are systematically identified and treated across specialties, including within general practice. Implementing computerized alerts for QRS duration and left ventricular (LV) function across both secondary and primary care levels could improve patient identification and treatment rates [121].

12. Conclusion and future directions

The journey of cardiac resynchronization therapy (CRT) from its nascent experimental stages to a well-established treatment for heart failure with reduced ejection fraction and ventricular dyssynchrony has been remarkable. CRT has undoubtedly changed the landscape of heart failure management, reducing symptoms, improving quality of life, and enhancing survival rates [122]. As evidenced by the CORE trials and other pivotal studies, CRT's utility in reversing negative remodeling and promoting a more efficient cardiac function is clear.

However, the path ahead is paved with challenges and opportunities that beckon further exploration. Future directions for the advancement of CRT include:

Personalization of therapy: Ongoing research aims to refine patient selection criteria through genetic profiling, advanced imaging techniques, and biometric data analysis to predict CRT response more accurately. Personalizing therapy may involve adjusting device settings and pacing strategies for individual patient anatomy and physiology.

Technological innovation: The development of leadless and modular CRT devices offers a glimpse into a future with minimally invasive procedures and reduced complications. Advances in battery technology, device miniaturization, and biocompatibility are expected to further improve patient outcomes and comfort.

Algorithm enhancement: Device-based algorithms that adapt to physiological changes in real-time and dynamically manage pacing are under investigation. These algorithms may potentially cater to daily variations in patient activity and circadian rhythms.

Combination therapies: Research into the synergistic effects of combining CRT with other heart failure therapies, such as novel pharmacological agents or stem cell therapy, could provide a multipronged approach to treating the underlying pathology of heart dysfunction.

Conduction system pacing: The exploration of pacing techniques that more closely mimic the heart's natural conduction system, such as His-bundle pacing or left bundle branch pacing, offers the promise of improved outcomes over traditional CRT.

Global accessibility: Efforts to increase the global accessibility of CRT, especially in low- and middle-income countries, are essential. This includes the development of cost-effective devices and training programs for local healthcare professionals.

Long-term studies: There is a need for long-term studies to understand the enduring impacts of CRT on chronic heart failure and to identify any late-emerging benefits or complications associated with therapy. In conclusion, while CRT has established itself as a cornerstone therapy for a subset of heart failure patients, the quest for optimization and innovation continues. Embracing a multidisciplinary approach that integrates advancements in technology, a deeper understanding of cardiac physiology, and individualized patient care is the key to unlocking the full potential of CRT in the future.

Thanks

To my parents, Alyah and Mohammed, my guiding stars in memory, whose love and wisdom resonate in every word.

Author details

Abdulmohsen Almusaad[1,2*], Muneera AlTaweel[2,3], Abdulrahman Abdullatif Alarfaj[4], Abdullah Dhawi Al-Otaibi[5], Mareyah Alshaikh Husain[6], Rasmah Saad Alharajin[4], Zainab Albahrani[7], Yousef Alanazi[7], Faisal Rabeea Alananzi[5], Sarah AlMukhaylid[8] and Ahmed Bander Alsalem[9]

1 King Abdulaziz Cardiac Center, King Abdulaziz Medical City, MNGHA, Riyadh, Saudi Arabia

2 King Abdullah International Medical Research Center (KAIMRC), Riyadh, Saudi Arabia

3 Department of Internal Medicine, King Abdulaziz Hospital, MNGHA, Riyadh, Al-Ahsa, Saudi Arabia

4 Family Medicine Department, King Abdulaziz National Guards Hospital, University Health Center, King Saud Bin Abdulaziz University for Health Sciences, Ministry of National Guard, Riyadh, Al-Ahsa, Saudi Arabia

5 Adult Cardiology Fellowship Training Program, Cardiac Sciences, King Abdulaziz Cardiac Center, King Abdulaziz Medical City, Ministry of National Guard Health Affairs, Riyadh, Saudi Arabia

6 Family Medicine Department, King Abdulaziz Hospital, NGHA, Al-Ahsa, Saudi Arabia

7 Department of Medicine, King Abdulaziz Hospital, MNGHA, Riyadh, Al-Ahsa, Saudi Arabia

8 College of Applied Medical Sciences (CoAMS-A), King Saud Bin Abdulaziz University for Health Sciences, Al-Mubarraz, Al-Ahsa, Saudi Arabia

9 College of Medicine, King Saud Bin Abdulaziz University for Health Sciences, King Abdulaziz Cardiac Center, National Guard Health Affairs, Riyadh, Saudi Arabia

*Address all correspondence to: a_almusaad@yahoo.com

References

[1] Yancy CW, Jessup M, Bozkurt B, Butler J, Casey DE Jr, Drazner MH, et al. 2013 ACCF/AHA guideline for the management of heart failure: A report of the American college of cardiology foundation/American heart association task force on practice guidelines. Circulation. 2013;**128**:240-327. DOI: 10.1161/cir.0b013e31829e8776

[2] Mehta VS, Elliott MK, Sidhu BS, Gould J, Porter B, Niederer S, et al. Multipoint pacing for cardiac resynchronisation therapy in patients with heart failure: A systematic review and meta-analysis. Journal of Cardiovascular Electrophysiology. 2021;**32**:2577-2589. DOI: 10.1111/jce.15199

[3] Sharma PS, Vijayaraman P. Conduction system pacing for cardiac resynchronisation. Arrhythmia & Electrophysiology Review. 2021;**10**:51-58. DOI: 0.15420/aer.2020.45

[4] Seriwala HM, Khan MS, Munir MB, Riaz IB, Riaz H, Saba S, et al. Leadless pacemakers: A new era in cardiac pacing. Journal of Cardiology. 2016;**67**:1-5. DOI: 10.1016/j.jjcc.2015.09.006

[5] Jafferani A, Leal M. Advances in cardiac resynchronization therapy. Journal of Innovations in Cardiac Rhythm Management. 2019;**10**:3681-3693. DOI: 10.19102/icrm.2019.100604

[6] Edafe EA, Iseko II, Dodiyi-Manuel ST. Cardiac resynchronization therapy: A 4-year review of our experience. International Journal of Innovative Research in Medical Science. 2022;7:699-702. DOI: 10.23958/ijirms/vol07-i12/1552

[7] Wiggers CJ. The muscular reactions of the mammalian ventricles to artificial surface stimuli. The American Journal of Physiology. 1925;**73**:346-378. DOI: 10.1152/ajplegacy.1925.73.2.346

[8] Strik M, Ploux S, Vernooy K, Prinzen FW. Cardiac resynchronization therapy—Refocus on the electrical substrate. Circulation Journal. 2011;**75**:1297-1304. DOI: 10.1253/circj.cj-11-0356

[9] Grines CL, Bashore TM, Boudoulas H, Olson S, Shafer P, Wooley CF. Functional abnormalities in isolated left bundle branch block. The effect of interventricular asynchrony. Circulation. 1989;**79**:845-853. DOI: 10.1161/01.cir.79.4.845

[10] Befeler B, Berkovits BV, Aranda JM, Sung RJ, Moleiro F, Castellanos A. Programmed simultaneous biventricular stimulation in man, with special reference to its use in the evaluation of intraventricular reentry. European Journal of Cardiology. 1979;**9**:369-378

[11] de Teresa E, Chamorro JL, Pulpón LA, Ruiz C, Bailón IR, Alzueta J, et al. An Even more Physiological Pacing: Changing the Sequence of Ventricular Activation. Cardiac Pacing, Heidelberg: Steinkopff; 1983. pp. 395-400

[12] Acena M, Regoli F, Auricchio A. Cardiac resynchronization therapy. Indications and contraindications. Revista Española de Cardiología (English Edition). 2012;**65**:843-849. DOI: 10.1016/j.rec.2012.02.026

[13] Bakker PF, Meijburg HW, de Vries JW, Mower MM, Thomas AC, Hull ML, et al. Biventricular pacing in end-stage heart failure improves functional capacity and left ventricular function. Journal of Interventional

Cardiac Electrophysiology. 2000;**4**:395-404. DOI: 10.1023/a:1009854417694

[14] Cazeau S, Ritter P, Bakdach S, Lazarus A, Limousin M, Henao L, et al. Four chamber pacing in dilated cardiomyopathy. Pacing and Clinical Electrophysiology. 1994;**17**:1974-1979. DOI: 10.1111/j.1540-8159.1994.tb03783.x

[15] Leclercq C, Gras D, Le Helloco A, Nicol L, Mabo P, Daubert C. Hemodynamic importance of preserving the normal sequence of ventricular activation in permanent cardiac pacing. American Heart Journal. 1995;**129**:1133-1141. DOI: 10.1016/0002-8703(95)90394-1

[16] Auricchio A, Klein H, Tockman B, Sack S, Stellbrink C, Neuzner J, et al. Transvenous biventricular pacing for heart failure: Can the obstacles be overcome? The American Journal of Cardiology. 1999;**83**:136-142. DOI: 10.1016/s0002-9149(98)01015-7

[17] Zipes DP, Jalife J, Stevenson WG. Cardiac Electrophysiology: From Cell to Bedside. 8th ed. Philadelphia, PA: Elsevier - Health Sciences Division; 2021

[18] Cheng A, Helm RH, Abraham TP. Pathophysiological mechanisms underlying ventricular dyssynchrony. Europace. 2009;**11**:v10-v14. DOI: 10.1093/europace/eup272

[19] Bogaert J, Rademakers FE. Dyssynchrony in heart failure: Mechanisms and clinical implications. Nature Reviews Cardiology. 2014;**11**(11):671-684

[20] Chung MK, Patton KK, Lau C-P, Dal Forno ARJ, Al-Khatib SM, Arora V, et al. 2023 HRS/APHRS/LAHRS guideline on cardiac physiologic pacing for the avoidance and mitigation of heart failure. Heart Rhythm. 2023;**20**:e17-e91. DOI: 10.1016/j.hrthm.2023.03.1538

[21] Wiegerinck RF, Schreurs R, Prinzen FW. Pathophysiology of dyssynchrony: Of squirrels and broken bones. Netherlands Heart Journal. 2016;**24**:4-10. DOI: 10.1007/s12471-015-0765-7

[22] Prinzen FW, Vernooy K, Auricchio A. Cardiac resynchronization therapy: State-of-the-art of current applications, guidelines, ongoing trials, and areas of controversy. Circulation. 2013;**128**:2407-2418. DOI: 10.1161/circulationaha.112.000112

[23] Rumsfeld JM, Kass DA. Cardiac resynchronization therapy: A comprehensive review of the evidence and guidelines. Journal of the American Medical Association. 2013;**309**(6):609-618. DOI: 10.1001/jama.2013.243

[24] Moss AJ, Hall WJ, Cannom DS, Klein H, Brown MW, Daubert JP, et al. Cardiac-resynchronization therapy for the prevention of heart-failure events. The New England Journal of Medicine. 2009;**361**:1329-1338. DOI: 10.1056/nejmoa0906431

[25] Crawford MH, Adams DH. Mitral valve regurgitation in heart failure: Pathophysiology, clinical implications, and management. Circulation. 2015;**131**(16):1436-1450. DOI: 10.1161/CIRCULATIONAHA.114.012216

[26] Boersma AK, Voors AA. Cellular and molecular mechanisms of cardiac resynchronization therapy. Nature Reviews Cardiology. 2014;**11**(11):665-675. DOI: 10.1038/nrcardio.2014.126

[27] Bristow MR, O'Connor CM. Energy metabolism in heart failure: Implications for cardiac resynchronization therapy. Journal of the American College of Cardiology. 2014;**64**(16):1723-1733. DOI: 10.1016/j.jacc.2014.07.083

[28] Cleland JGF, Daubert J-C, Erdmann E, Freemantle N, Gras D, Kappenberger L, et al. The effect of cardiac resynchronization on morbidity and mortality in heart failure. The New England Journal of Medicine. 2005;**352**:1539-1549. DOI: 10.1056/nejmoa050496

[29] Abraham WT, Fisher WG, Smith AL, Delurgio DB, Leon AR, Loh E, et al. Cardiac resynchronization in chronic heart failure. The New England Journal of Medicine. 2002;**346**:1845-1853. DOI: 10.1056/nejmoa013168

[30] Moss AJ, Zareba W, Hall WJ, Klein H, Wilber DJ, Cannom DS, et al. Prophylactic implantation of a defibrillator in patients with myocardial infarction and reduced ejection fraction. The New England Journal of Medicine. 2002;**346**:877-883. DOI: 10.1056/nejmoa013474

[31] Kadish A, Dyer A, Daubert JP, Friedman PA, Greene HL, Gregoratos G, et al. Cardiac resynchronization and defibrillation in heart failure. The New England Journal of Medicine. 2004;**350**:2528-2537

[32] Anand IS, Carson P, Galle E, Song R, Boehmer J, Ghali JK, et al. Cardiac resynchronization therapy reduces the risk of hospitalizations in patients with advanced Heart Failure: Results from the Comparison of Medical Therapy, Pacing and Defibrillation in Heart Failure (COMPANION) trial. Circulation. 2009;**119**:969-977. DOI: 10.1161/circulationaha.108.793273

[33] Bristow MR, Saxon LA, Boehmer J, Krueger S, Kass DA, De Marco T, et al. Cardiac-resynchronization therapy with or without an implantable defibrillator in advanced chronic heart failure. The New England Journal of Medicine. 2004;**350**:2140-2150. DOI: 10.1056/nejmoa032423

[34] Leclercq C, Burri H, Delnoy PP, Rinaldi CA, Sperzel J, Calò L, et al. Cardiac resynchronization therapy non-responder to responder conversion rate in the MORE-CRT MPP trial. Europace. 2023;**25**:euad294. DOI: 10.1093/europace/euad294

[35] St John Sutton MG, Plappert T, Abraham WT, Smith AL, DeLurgio DB, Leon AR, et al. Effect of cardiac resynchronization therapy on left ventricular size and function in chronic heart failure. Circulation. 2003;**107**:1985-1990. DOI: 10.1161/01.cir.0000065226.24159.e9

[36] Tang ASL, Wells GA, Talajic M, Arnold MO, Sheldon R, Connolly S, et al. Cardiac-resynchronization therapy for mild-to-moderate heart failure. The New England Journal of Medicine. 2010;**363**:2385-2395. DOI: 10.1056/nejmoa1009540

[37] Sohaib SMA, Finegold JA, Nijjer SS, Hossain R, Linde C, Levy WC, et al. Opportunity to increase life span in narrow QRS cardiac resynchronization therapy recipients by deactivating ventricular pacing. JACC: Heart Failure. 2015;**3**:327-336. DOI: 10.1016/j.jchf.2014.11.007

[38] Healey JS, Hohnloser SH, Exner DV, Birnie DH, Parkash R, Connolly SJ, et al. Cardiac resynchronization therapy in patients with permanent atrial fibrillation: Results from the Resynchronization for Ambulatory Heart Failure Trial (RAFT). Circulation. Heart Failure. 2012;**5**:566-570. DOI: 10.1161/circheartfailure.112.968867

[39] Lopes C, Pereira T, Barra S. Cardiac resynchronization therapy in patients with atrial fibrillation: A meta-analysis. Revista Portuguesa de Cardiologia. 2014;**33**:717-725. DOI: 10.1016/j.repc.2014.05.008

[40] Upadhyay GA, Choudhry NK, Auricchio A, Ruskin J, Singh JP. Cardiac resynchronization in patients with atrial fibrillation. Journal of the American College of Cardiology. 2008;**52**:1239-1246. DOI: 10.1016/j.jacc.2008.06.043

[41] Elliott MK, Mehta VS, Martic D, Sidhu BS, Niederer S, Rinaldi CA. Atrial fibrillation in cardiac resynchronization therapy. Heart Rhythm O2. 2021;**2**:784-795. DOI: 10.1016/j.hroo.2021.09.003

[42] Jaffe LM, Morin DP. Cardiac resynchronization therapy: History, present status, and future directions. The Ochsner Journal. 2014;**14**:596-607

[43] Khurwolah MR, Yao J, Kong X-Q. Adverse consequences of Right Ventricular Apical pacing and novel strategies to optimize Left Ventricular systolic and diastolic function. Current Cardiology Reviews. 2019;**15**:145-155. DOI: 10.2174/1573403x15666181129161839

[44] Jankelson L, Bordachar P, Strik M, Ploux S, Chinitz L. Reducing right ventricular pacing burden: Algorithms, benefits, and risks. Europace. 2019;**21**:539-547. DOI: 10.1093/europace/euy263

[45] Das A, Kahali D. Ventricular septal pacing: Optimum method to position the lead. Indian Heart Journal. 2018;**70**:713-720. DOI: 10.1016/j.ihj.2018.01.023

[46] Brignole M, Pentimalli F, Palmisano P, Landolina M, Quartieri F, Occhetta E, et al. AV junction ablation and cardiac resynchronization for patients with permanent atrial fibrillation and narrow QRS: The APAF-CRT mortality trial. European Heart Journal. 2021;**42**:4731-4739. DOI: 10.1093/eurheartj/ehab569

[47] Curtis AB, Worley SJ, Adamson PB, Chung ES, Niazi I, Sherfesee L, et al. Biventricular pacing for atrioventricular block and systolic dysfunction. The New England Journal of Medicine. 2013;**368**:1585-1593. DOI: 10.1056/nejmoa1210356

[48] Yu C-M, Chan JY-S, Zhang Q, Omar R, Yip GW-K, Hussin A, et al. Biventricular pacing in patients with bradycardia and normal ejection fraction. The New England Journal of Medicine. 2009;**361**:2123-2134. DOI: 10.1056/nejmoa0907555

[49] Fang F, Sanderson JE, Yu C-M. Should all patients with heart block receive biventricular pacing?: All heart block patients with a pacemaker indication should receive biventricular pacing: One move, double the gains? Circulation. Arrhythmia and Electrophysiology. 2015;**8**:722-729. DOI: 10.1161/circep.114.000626

[50] Ellenbogen KA, Auricchio A, Burri H, Gold MR, Leclercq C, Leyva F, et al. The evolving state of cardiac resynchronization therapy and conduction system pacing: 25 years of research at EP Europace journal. Europace. 2023;**25**:euad168. DOI: 10.1093/europace/euad168

[51] Leyva F, Zegard A, Umar F, Taylor RJ, Acquaye E, Gubran C, et al. Long-term clinical outcomes of cardiac resynchronization therapy with or without defibrillation: Impact of the aetiology of cardiomyopathy. Europace. 2018;**20**:1804-1812. DOI: 10.1093/europace/eux357

[52] Dan G-A. 2021 ESC guidelines on cardiac pacing and cardiac resynchronisation therapy. European Cardiology Review. 2021;**16**:3427-3520. DOI: 10.15420/ecr.2021.51

[53] Singh JP, Cha YM, Lunati M, Chung ES, Li S, Smeets P, O'Donnell D.

Real-world behavior of CRT pacing using the AdaptivCRT algorithm on patient outcomes: Effect on mortality and atrial fibrillation incidence. Journal of Cardiovascular Electrophysiology. Apr 2020;**31**(4):825-833. DOI: 10.1111/jce.14376

[54] Tan L, Ganesananthan S, Huzaien H, Elsayed H, Shah N, Shah P, et al. Upgrading to cardiac resynchronisation therapy: Concordance of real-world experience with clinical guidelines. International Journal of Cardiology. Heart & vasculature. 2021;**33**:100746. DOI: 10.1016/j.ijcha.2021.100746

[55] Heidenreich PA, Bozkurt B, Aguilar D, Allen LA, Byun JJ, Colvin MM, et al. 2022 ACC/AHA/HFSA guideline for the management of heart failure. Journal of Cardiac Failure. 2022;**28**:e1-e167. DOI: 10.1016/j.cardfail.2022.02.010

[56] Strauss DG, Jais P, Hocini M, et al. Left bundle branch block: Time for a new definition? Heart. 2016;**102**:754-760. DOI: 10.1136/heartjnl-2015-308718

[57] Simon A, Pilecky D, Kiss LZ, Vamos M. Useful electrocardiographic signs to support the prediction of favorable response to cardiac resynchronization therapy. Journal of Cardiovascular Development and Disease. 2023;**10**:425. DOI: 10.3390/jcdd10100425

[58] Ponikowski P, Voors AA, Anker SD, Bueno H, Cleland JGF, Coats AJS, et al. 2016 ESC Guidelines for the diagnosis and treatment of acute and chronic heart failure: The Task Force for the diagnosis and treatment of acute and chronic heart failure of the European Society of Cardiology (ESC) Developed with the special contribution of the Heart Failure Association (HFA) of the ESC. European Heart Journal. 2016;**37**:2129-2200

[59] Zipes DP, Camm AJ, Borggrefe M, Buxton AE, Chaitman B, Fromer M, et al. ACC/AHA/ESC 2006 guidelines for management of patients with ventricular arrhythmias and the prevention of sudden cardiac death. Journal of the American College of Cardiology. 2006;**48**:e247-e346. DOI: 10.1016/j.jacc.2006.07.010

[60] Hohnloser SH, Kuck KH, Dorian P, et al. Effect of metoprolol CR/XL in chronic heart failure with reduced ejection fraction: A double-blind, placebo-controlled trial. Lancet. 2002;**36**:1349-1355. DOI: 10.1016/S0140-6736(02)11456-5

[61] Van Stipdonk MJ, Sacher F, Verouden NJ, et al. Impact of left bundle branch block criteria on electrocardiographic and clinical characteristics of cardiac resynchronization therapy patients: A multicenter study. Journal of the American College of Cardiology. 2015;**65**(13):1315-1323. DOI: 10.1016/j.jacc.2015.01.039

[62] Thibault B, Harel F, Ducharme A, White M, Ellenbogen KA, Frasure-Smith N, et al. Cardiac Resynchronization Therapy in patients with Heart Failure and a QRS complex <120 milliseconds: The Evaluation of Resynchronization Therapy for Heart Failure (LESSER-EARTH) trial. Circulation. 2013;**127**:873-881. DOI: 10.1161/circulationaha.112.001239

[63] Ruschitzka F, Abraham WT, Singh JP, Bax JJ, Borer JS, Brugada J, et al. Cardiac-resynchronization therapy in heart failure with a narrow QRS complex. The New England Journal of Medicine. 2013;**369**:1395-1405. DOI: 10.1056/nejmoa1306687

[64] Moskovitch J, Voskoboinik A. Cardiac resynchronization therapy: A

comprehensive review. Minerva Medica. 2019;**110**:121-138. DOI: 10.23736/s0026-4806.18.05861-5

[65] Sieniewicz BJ, Gould J, Porter B, Sidhu BS, Teall T, Webb J, et al. Understanding non-response to cardiac resynchronisation therapy: Common problems and potential solutions. Heart Failure Reviews. 2019;**24**:41-54. DOI: 10.1007/s10741-018-9734-8

[66] Wang Y, Sharbaugh MS, Munir MB, Adelstein EC, Wang NC, Althouse AD, et al. Gender differences in cardiac resynchronization therapy device choice and outcome in patients ≥75 years of age with heart failure. The American Journal of Cardiology. 2017;**120**:2201-2206. DOI: 10.1016/j.amjcard.2017.08.044

[67] Poposka L, Boskov V, Risteski D, Taleski J, Janusevski F, Srbinovska E, et al. Electrocardiographic parameters as predictors of response to cardiac resynchronization therapy. Open Access Macedonian Journal of Medical Sciences. 2018;**6**:297-302. DOI: 10.3889/oamjms.2018.092

[68] Bax JJ et al. ECG variables: (S1 + R6) − (S6 + R1). Heart Rhythm. 2018;**15**(12):1851-1858

[69] Gupta D et al. R6/S6 ratio. Journal of Electrocardiology. 2017;**50**(6):721-727

[70] Kapoor A et al. Height of R wave in V6. Indian Heart Journal. 2016;**68**(6):741-747

[71] Auricchio A et al. LBBB vs. non-LBBB patients. European Heart Journal. 2015;**36**(38):2627-2635

[72] Yu C-M, Sanderson JE, Gorcsan J. Echocardiography, dyssynchrony, and the response to cardiac resynchronization therapy. European Heart Journal. 2010;**31**:2326-2337. DOI: 10.1093/eurheartj/ehq263

[73] Owen JS, Khatib S, Morin DP. Cardiac resynchronization therapy. The Ochsner Journal. 2009;**9**:248

[74] Gosling RC, Al-Mohammad A. The role of cardiac imaging in heart failure with reduced ejection fraction. Cardiac Failure Review. 24 Jun 2022;**8**:e22. DOI: 10.15420/cfr.2021.33

[75] Galli E, Galand V, Le Rolle V, Taconne M, Wazzan AA, Hernandez A, et al. The saga of dyssynchrony imaging: Are we getting to the point. Frontiers in Cardiovascular Medicine. 31 March 2023;**10**. DOI: 10.3389/fcvm.2023.1111538

[76] Leyva F, Nisam S, Auricchio A. 20 years of cardiac resynchronization therapy. Journal of the American College of Cardiology. 2014;**64**:1047-1058. DOI: 10.1016/j.jacc.2014.06.1178

[77] Writing Committee Members, Epstein AE, DiMarco JP, Ellenbogen KA, Estes NAM III, Freedman RA, et al. ACC/AHA/HRS 2008 guidelines for device-based therapy of cardiac rhythm abnormalities: A report of the American college of cardiology/American heart association task force on practice guidelines (writing committee to revise the ACC/AHA/NASPE 2002 guideline update for implantation of cardiac pacemakers and antiarrhythmia devices): Developed in collaboration with the American association for thoracic surgery and society of thoracic surgeons. Circulation. **2008;117**:e350-e408. DOI: 10.1161/circualtionaha.108.189742

[78] Cazeau S, Leclercq C, Lavergne T, Walker S, Varma C, Linde C, et al. Effects of multisite biventricular pacing in patients with heart failure and intraventricular conduction delay. The New England Journal of Medicine. 2001;**344**:873-880. DOI: 10.1056/nejm200103223441202

[79] Gold MR, Birgersdotter-Green U, Singh JP, Ellenbogen KA, Yu Y, Meyer TE, et al. The relationship between ventricular electrical delay and left ventricular remodelling with cardiac resynchronization therapy. European Heart Journal. 2011;**32**:2516-2524. DOI: 10.1093/eurheartj/ehr329

[80] Becker M, Kramann R, Franke A, Breithardt O-A, Heussen N, Knackstedt C, et al. Impact of left ventricular lead position in cardiac resynchronization therapy on left ventricular remodelling. A circumferential strain analysis based on 2D echocardiography. European Heart Journal. 2007;**28**:1211-1220. DOI: 10.1093/eurheartj/ehm034

[81] Saba S, Marek J, Schwartzman D, Jain S, Adelstein E, White P, et al. Echocardiography-guided left ventricular lead placement for cardiac resynchronization therapy: Results of the Speckle Tracking Assisted Resynchronization Therapy for Electrode Region trial. Circulation. Heart Failure. 2013;**6**:427-434. DOI: 10.1161/circheartfailure.112.000078

[82] Leyva F. Cardiac resynchronization therapy guided by cardiovascular magnetic resonance. Journal of Cardiovascular Magnetic Resonance. 2010;**12**:64. DOI: 10.1186/1532-429x-12-64

[83] Massacesi C, Ceriello L, Maturo F, Porreca A, Appignani M, Di Girolamo E. Cardiac resynchronization therapy with multipoint pacing via quadripolar lead versus traditional biventricular pacing: A systematic review and meta-analysis of clinical studies on hemodynamic, clinical, and prognostic parameters. Heart Rhythm O2. 2021;**2**:682-690. DOI: 10.1016/j.hroo.2021.09.012

[84] Almusaad A, Sweidan R, Alanazi H, Jamiel A, Bokhari F, Al Hebaishi Y, et al. Long-term reverse remodeling and clinical improvement by Multi Point Pacing in a randomized, international, Middle Eastern heart failure study. Journal of Interventional Cardiac Electrophysiology. 2022;**63**:399-407. DOI: 10.1007/s10840-020-00928-2

[85] Lunati M, Magenta G, Cattafi G, Moreo A, Falaschi G, Contardi D, et al. Clinical relevance of systematic CRT device optimization. Journal of Atrial Fibrillation. 2014;7:1077. DOI: 10.4022/jafib.1077

[86] Schiavone M, Arosio R, Valenza S, Ruggiero D, Mitacchione G, Lombardi L, et al. Cardiac resynchronization therapy: Present and future. European Heart Journal Supplements: Journal of the European Society of Cardiology. 2023;**25**:C227-C233. DOI: 10.1093/eurheartjsupp/suad046

[87] Narula OS, Scherlag BJ, Samet P. Pervenous pacing of the specialized conducting system in man: His bundle and A-V nodal stimulation. Circulation. 1970;**41**:77-87. DOI: 10.1161/01.cir.41.1.77

[88] Zhang J, Guo J, Hou X, Wang Y, Qian Z, Li K, et al. Comparison of the effects of selective and non-selective His bundle pacing on cardiac electrical and mechanical synchrony. Europace. 2018;**20**:1010-1017. DOI: 10.1093/europace/eux120

[89] Deshmukh P, Casavant DA, Romanyshyn M, Anderson K. Permanent, Direct His-bundle pacing: A novel approach to cardiac pacing in patients with normal His-Purkinje activation. Circulation. 2000;**101**:869-877. DOI: 10.1161/01.cir.101.8.869

[90] Upadhyay GA, Vijayaraman P, Nayak HM, Verma N, Dandamudi G, Sharma PS, et al. On-treatment comparison between corrective His

bundle pacing and biventricular pacing for cardiac resynchronization: A secondary analysis of the His-SYNC Pilot Trial. Heart Rhythm. 2019;**16**:1797-1807. DOI: 10.1016/j.hrthm.2019.05.009

[91] Vinther M, Risum N, Svendsen JH, Møgelvang R, Philbert BT. A randomized trial of His pacing versus biventricular pacing in symptomatic HF patients with left bundle branch block (His-alternative). JACC: Clinical Electrophysiology. 2021;**7**:1422-1432. DOI: 10.1016/j.jacep.2021.04.003

[92] Ivanovski M, Zupan Mežnar A, Štublar J, Žižek D. His bundle pacing: Initial Slovenian single-Centre experience. Slovenian Medical Journal. 2021;**90**:587-595. DOI: 10.6016/zdravvestn.3196

[93] Rijks J, Luermans J, Heckman L, van Stipdonk AMW, Prinzen F, Lumens J, et al. Physiology of left ventricular septal pacing and left bundle branch pacing. Cardiac Electrophysiology Clinics. 2022;**14**:181-189. DOI: 10.1016/j.ccep.2021.12.010

[94] Vijayaraman P, Naperkowski A, Subzposh FA, Abdelrahman M, Sharma PS, Oren JW, et al. Permanent His-bundle pacing: Long-term lead performance and clinical outcomes. Heart Rhythm. 2018;**15**:696-702. DOI: 10.1016/j.hrthm.2017.12.022

[95] Vijayaraman P, Herweg B, Verma A, Sharma PS, Batul SA, Ponnusamy SS, et al. Rescue left bundle branch area pacing in coronary venous lead failure or nonresponse to biventricular pacing: Results from International LBBAP Collaborative Study Group. Heart Rhythm. 2022;**19**:1272-1280. DOI: 10.1016/j.hrthm.2022.04.024

[96] Curila K, Jurak P, Jastrzebski M, Prinzen F, Waldauf P, Halamek J, et al. Left bundle branch pacing compared to left ventricular septal myocardial pacing increases interventricular dyssynchrony but accelerates left ventricular lateral wall depolarization. Heart Rhythm. 2021;**18**:1281-1289. DOI: 10.1016/j.hrthm.2021.04.025

[97] Liu J, Sun F, Wang Z, Sun J, Jiang X, Zhao W, et al. Left bundle branch area pacing vs. biventricular pacing for cardiac resynchronization therapy: A meta-analysis. Frontiers in Cardiovascular Medicine. 24 May 2021;**8**. DOI: 10.3389/fcvm.2021.669301

[98] Diaz JC, Tedrow UB, Duque M, Aristizabal J, Braunstein ED, Marin J, et al. Left bundle branch pacing vs left ventricular septal pacing vs biventricular pacing for cardiac resynchronization therapy. JACC: Clinical Electrophysiology. Feb 2024;**10**(2):295-305. DOI: 10.1016/j.jacep.2023.10.016

[99] Salden FCWM, Luermans JGLM, Westra SW, Weijs B, Engels EB, Heckman LIB, et al. Short-term hemodynamic and electrophysiological effects of cardiac resynchronization by left ventricular septal pacing. Journal of the American College of Cardiology. 2020;**75**:347-359. DOI: 10.1016/j.jacc.2019.11.040

[100] Huang W, Su L, Wu S, Xu L, Xiao F, Zhou X, et al. A novel pacing strategy with low and stable output: Pacing the left bundle branch immediately beyond the conduction block. The Canadian Journal of Cardiology. 2017;**33**:1736.e1-1736.e3. DOI: 10.1016/j.cjca.2017.09.013

[101] De Pooter J, Calle S, Timmermans F, Van Heuverswyn F. Left bundle branch area pacing using stylet-driven pacing leads with a new delivery sheath: A comparison with lumen-less leads. Journal of Cardiovascular

Electrophysiology. 2021;**32**:439-448. DOI: 10.1111/jce.14851

[102] Huang W, Chen X, Su L, Wu S, Xia X, Vijayaraman P. A beginner's guide to permanent left bundle branch pacing. Heart Rhythm. 2019;**16**:1791-1796. DOI: 10.1016/j.hrthm.2019.06.016

[103] Qi P, Li X-X, Tian Y, Shi L, Wang Y-J, Liu X-P. Injection of contrast medium through a delivery sheath reveals interventricular septal vascular injury in a case of left bundle branch pacing. The Journal of International Medical Research. 2020;**48**:030006052094788. DOI: 10.1177/0300060520947880

[104] Elliott MK, Mehta VS, Sidhu BS, Niederer S, Rinaldi CA. Endocardial left ventricular pacing. Herz. 2021;**46**:526-532. DOI: 10.1007/s00059-021-05074-7

[105] Mendonca Costa C, Neic A, Gillette K, Porter B, Gould J, Sidhu B, et al. Left ventricular endocardial pacing is less arrhythmogenic than conventional epicardial pacing when pacing in proximity to scar. Heart Rhythm. 2020;**17**:1262-1270. DOI: 10.1016/j.hrthm.2020.03.021

[106] Veenis JF, Brunner-La Rocca H-P, Linssen GCM, Geerlings PR, Van Gent MWF, Aksoy I, et al. Age differences in contemporary treatment of patients with chronic heart failure and reduced ejection fraction. European Journal of Preventive Cardiology. 2019;**26**:1399-1407. DOI: 10.1177/2047487319835042

[107] Reddy VY, Miller MA, Neuzil P, Søgaard P, Butter C, Seifert M, et al. Cardiac resynchronization therapy with wireless left ventricular endocardial pacing. Journal of the American College of Cardiology. 2017;**69**:2119-2129. DOI: 10.1016/j.jacc.2017.02.059

[108] Sidhu BS, Gould J, Elliott MK, Mehta V, Niederer S, Rinaldi CA. Leadless left ventricular endocardial pacing and left bundle branch area pacing for cardiac resynchronisation therapy. Arrhythmia & Electrophysiology Review. 2021;**10**:45-50. DOI: 10.15420/aer.2020.46

[109] Task Force Chairs, Daubert J-C, Saxon L, Adamson PB, Auricchio A, Berger RD, et al. 2012 EHRA/HRS expert consensus statement on cardiac resynchronization therapy in heart failure: Implant and follow-up recommendations and management: A registered branch of the European Society of Cardiology (ESC), and the Heart Rhythm Society; and in collaboration with the Heart Failure Society of America (HFSA), the American Society of Echocardiography (ASE), the American Heart Association (AHA), the European Association of Echocardiography (EAE) of the ESC and the Heart Failure Association of the ESC (HFA). * Endorsed by the governing bodies of AHA, ASE, EAE, HFSA, HFA, EHRA, and HRS. Europace. 2012;**14**:1236-1286. DOI: 10.1093/europace/eus222

[110] Merkely B, Molnar L, Rok A. Interventional and minimally invasive surgical techniques facilitating cardiac resynchronization therapy. In: Roka A, editor. Current Issues and Recent Advances in Pacemaker Therapy. London, England: InTech; 2012. DOI: 10.5772/50291

[111] Lee CK, Yoo SY, Hong MY, Jang JK. Antithrombotic or anti-platelet agents in patients undergoing permanent pacemaker implantation. Korean Circulation Journal. 2012;**42**:538. DOI: 10.4070/kcj.2012.42.8.538

[112] Hasdemir C. Cardiac resynchronization therapy: Implantation tips and tricks. Anadolu Kardiyoloji Dergisi. 2007;**7**(Suppl. 1):53-56

[113] Pothineni N, Gondi S, Cherian T, Kovelamudi S, Schaller R, Lakkireddy D, et al. Complications of cardiac resynchronization therapy: Comparison of safety outcomes from real-world studies and clinical trials. Journal of Innovations in Cardiac Rhythm Management. 2022;**13**:5121-5125. DOI: 10.19102/icrm.2022.130805

[114] Borgquist R, Barrington WR, Bakos Z, Werther-Evaldsson A, Saba S. Targeting the latest site of left ventricular mechanical activation is associated with improved long-term outcomes for recipients of cardiac resynchronization therapy. Heart Rhythm O2. 2022;**3**:377-384. DOI: 10.1016/j.hroo.2022.05.003

[115] Kutyifa V, Zareba W, McNitt S, Singh J, Hall WJ, Polonsky S, et al. Left ventricular lead location and the risk of ventricular arrhythmias in the MADIT-CRT trial. European Heart Journal. 2013;**34**:184-190. DOI: 10.1093/eurheartj/ehs334

[116] Butter C, Georgi C, Stockburger M. Optimal CRT implantation—Where and how to place the left-ventricular lead? Current Heart Failure Reports. 2021;**18**:329-344. DOI: 10.1007/s11897-021-00528-9

[117] Shepard RK, Ellenbogen KA. Challenges and solutions for difficult implantations of CRT devices: The role of new technology and techniques. Journal of Cardiovascular Electrophysiology. 2007;**18**(1):S21-S25. DOI: 10.1111/j.1540-8167.2007.00707.x

[118] Shah R, Qualls Z. Diaphragmatic stimulation caused by cardiac resynchronization treatment. CMAJ. 2016;**188**:E239-E239. DOI: 10.1503/cmaj.150986

[119] Curtis AB, Yancy CW, Albert NM, Stough WG, Gheorghiade M, Heywood JT, et al. Cardiac resynchronization therapy utilization for heart failure: Findings from IMPROVE HF. American Heart Journal. 2009;**158**:956-964. DOI: 10.1016/j.ahj.2009.10.011

[120] Foley PWX, Leyva F, Frenneaux MP. What is treatment success in cardiac resynchronization therapy? Europace. 2009;**11**:v58-v65. DOI: 10.1093/europace/eup308

[121] Gorodeski EZ, Magnelli-Reyes C, Moennich LA, Grimaldi A, Rickard J. Cardiac resynchronization therapy-heart failure (CRT-HF) clinic: A novel model of care. PLoS ONE. 2019;**14**:e0222610. DOI: 10.1371/journal.pone.0222610

[122] Pitzalis MV, Iacoviello M, Romito R, Massari F, Rizzon B, Luzzi G, et al. Cardiac resynchronization therapy tailored by echocardiographic evaluation of ventricular asynchrony. Journal of the American College of Cardiology. 2002;**40**:1615-1622. DOI: 10.1016/s0735-1097(02)02337-9

Chapter 4

A Comprehensive Approach to Cardiac Resynchronization Therapy

Malik Ghawanmeh, Dorys Chavez, Luis Cerna Urrutia and Cynthia M. Tracy

Abstract

This chapter aims to comprehensively examine and offer guidance on the contemporary indications for Cardiac Resynchronization Therapy (CRT) in individuals with pacemaker indications or heart failure. Herein we examine the contemporary understanding of CRT responders by analyzing the latest evidence. We explore the impact of CRT on mortality rates, heart failure hospitalizations, clinical parameters of heart failure, stabilization of ventricular function, and its role in preventing the progression of heart failure. We delve into the latest advancements in physiological pacing, encompassing anatomical and physiological characteristics, while critically evaluating the associated advantages and disadvantages. Additionally, the chapter explores future prospects and directions in the field, providing a well-rounded overview of the evolving landscape of CRT.

Keywords: conduction system pacing, cardiac physiologic pacing, cardiac resynchronization therapy, heart failure with reduced ejection fraction, left bundle branch block

1. Introduction

Cardiac Physiologic Pacing (CPP) is at the forefront of device management in Heart Failure with reduced Ejection Fraction (HFrEF). The 2023 HRS/APHRS/LAHRS guideline on Cardiac Physiologic Pacing for the avoidance and mitigation of heart failure defined CPP as "cardiac pacing intended to restore or preserve ventricular synchrony". CPP includes cardiac resynchronization therapy (CRT) and Conduction System Pacing (CSP). CRT uses left ventricular (LV) stimulation and Biventricular (BiV) pacing by utilizing a lead placed in a coronary sinus branch in the LV epicardium. CSP includes His bundle pacing (HBP), or left bundle branch area pacing (LBBAP). The evidence supporting CRT use in HFrEF is more robust than that of Conduction System Pacing (CSP) due to the longer duration of its widespread application [1]. The primary focus of this chapter is CRT: pathophysiology, indications, patient selection, procedural aspect, current evidence of CRT, and future CRT directions and innovation.

2. Pathophysiology of cardiac dyssynchrony

In the normal physiologic depolarization sequence, the initial electrical activation originates in the LV and Right Ventricular (RV) endocardium. This progression unfolds with the depolarization of the septum from left to right, followed by the swift activation of the remaining LV myocardium, including the lateral wall, through specialized conduction tissue [2].

Conversely, with left bundle branch block (LBBB), depolarization initiates in the right ventricular endocardium. Subsequently, septal activation occurs through impulses transmitted from the right bundle branch, moving in a right-to-left direction. This activation then traverses to the left ventricular endocardium, reaching and activating the remainder of the left ventricular myocardium. Notably, this latter route partially bypasses specialized conduction tissue, leading to a delayed activation of the lateral wall creating electromechanical dyssynchrony [3].

Electromechanical dyssynchrony caused by a LBBB carries significant hemodynamic implications, potentially resulting in diminished LV contraction and compromised relaxation. This can culminate in adverse remodeling over an extended period. Consequently, a subset of individuals experiencing prolonged LBBB may be susceptible to the development of dyssynchrony-induced cardiomyopathy, characterized by a reduction in left ventricular ejection fraction (LVEF) and the onset of heart failure (HF). Similarly, patients with high percentages of RV only pacing may develop dyssynchrony from a similar mechanism [4].

Acknowledging the reversible nature of electromechanical dyssynchrony-induced cardiomyopathy underscores the importance of routine assessments of ventricular function in the specific context of LBBB or high percentage RV pacing. The integration of tailored therapeutic approaches such as CRT can play a pivotal role in mitigating the impact of electrodyssynchrony [5].

3. Evidence

Prior to the MUSTIC (Multisite Stimulation in Cardiomyopathies) trial in 2001 and PATH-CHF (The Pacing Therapies for Congestive Heart Failure) trial in 2002, observational studies had highlighted the negative impact of RV pacing on heart failure patients and the positive hemodynamic changes in the pulmonary capillary wedge pressure and cardiac output [6]. Despite their limitations in sample size and study design, the MUSTIC and PATH-HF trials established the efficacy of CRT pacing in selected chronic systolic heart failure patients with intraventricular conduction delay and showcased positive outcomes such as improved walking distance and reduced HF hospitalizations (**Figure 1**) [8, 9].

These pivotal trials paved the way for the MIRACLE (Multicenter InSync Randomized Clinical Evaluation) study, the first double-blinded randomized clinical trial involving 453 patients with moderate to severe HF and QRS duration ≥130 ms. This trial validated the efficacy of CRT-P + Optimal Medical Therapy (OPT) compared to OPT alone. CRT-P + OPT combination reduced NYHA functional class and HF hospitalization in addition to improving quality of life and LVEF [10]. This was followed by the MIRACLE ICD study involving 369 patients with moderate to severe HF and QRS duration ≥130 ms. This trial demonstrated the safety and efficacy of combined CRT and ICD therapy (CRT-D) compared to ICD therapy alone. CRT-D improves quality of life and functional class [11].

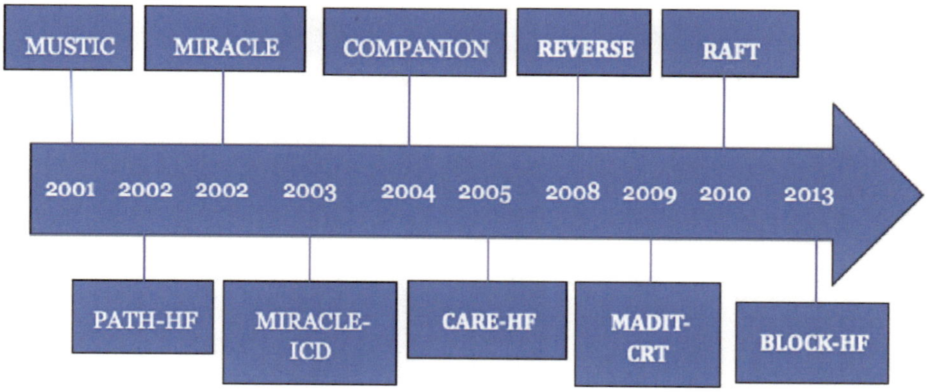

Figure 1.
A timeline of the core CRT clinical trials [7].

In 2004, the COMPANION (Comparison of Medical Therapy, Pacing and Defibrillation in Heart Failure) trial was the first randomized clinical trial to compare CRT-P and CRT-D + OPT to OPT alone. The primary composite endpoint, encompassing time to death from any cause or hospitalization, showed a decreased risk with both CRT-P (HR 0.81) and CRT-D (HR 0.80) compared to OPT alone [12]. Subsequently, in 2005, CARE-HF (Cardiac Resynchronization-Heart Failure) trial compared CRT + OPT to OPT alone in 813 patients. The findings were consistent with previous clinical trials: the primary endpoint, time to death from any cause or unplanned hospitalization for a major cardiovascular event, was lower in CRT group (39%) vs. OPT group (55%). The secondary endpoint of death from any cause was also lower in the CRT group (20% vs. 30%) [13].

The COMPANION and the CARE-HF landmark trials laid the foundation for using CRT-P and CRT-D as part of the Guideline Directed Medical Therapy (GDMT) in HFrEF (EF ≤35%) with NYHA class III-IV and wide QRS complex (≥120 ms).

The benefit of CRT in mild symptomatic HF was not fully explored until the publication of REVERSE (Resynchronization Reverses Remodeling in Systolic Left Ventricular Dysfunction) and MADIT-CRT (Multicenter Automatic Defibrillator Implantation Trial with Cardiac Resynchronization Therapy) trials in 2008 and 2009. The REVERSE randomized 610 patients with NYHA Class I-II, EF < 40% and wide QRS (≥120 ms) to active CRT vs. control. Active CRT in combination with medical therapy reduces HF hospitalization and improves the LV structure and function [14]. The MADIT-CRT randomized 1820 patients with NYHA Class I-II, EF < 30% and a wide QRS (≥130 ms) to CRT-D vs. ICD alone. CRT-D had HR 0.66, P = 0.001 in the primary endpoint (death or nonfatal heart-failure events) compared to ICD alone. CRT-D arm had 41% reduction in HF hospitalization especially with QRS duration >150 ms. CRT-D was also associated with improved LVEF and volumes [15].

The BLOCK HF (Biventricular versus Right Ventricular Pacing in Heart Failure Patients with Atrioventricular Block) study demonstrated the superiority of the BiV pacing over RV pacing only in patients with atrioventricular block, LVEF ≤50%, and NYHA Class I-II. The primary outcome was comprising death from any cause, an urgent care visit for heart failure requiring intravenous therapy, or a 15% or more increase in the left ventricular end-systolic volume index. The HR for the primary outcome was 0.74 suggesting the CRT role in mitigating adverse LV remodeling and improving overall outcomes compared to RV pacing only (**Table 1**) [16].

Trial name	Date	Sample Size	EF	QRS duration	NYHA class	Primary outcomes	Results
MUSTIC [8]	2001	48	≤35%	≥150 ms	III	Distance walked in six minutes, quality of life, peak oxygen consumption, hospitalizations related to heart failure, and mortality rate.	CRT-P improved walking distance and quality of life, reduced HF hospitalization
PATH-HF [9]	2002	41	NA	≥120 ms	III-IV	Oxygen uptake during bicycle exercise and the 6-minute walk distance	CRT-P improved walking distance and peak VO2 after 12 months
MIRACLE [10]	2002	571	≤35%	≥130 ms	III-IV	NYHA class, quality of life, and the distance walked in six minutes.	CRT-P improves six minutes walking distance, NYHA functional class, quality of life, time on the treadmill during exercise testing, and EF
MIRACLE ICD [11]	2003	369	≤35%	≥130 ms	III-IV	NYHA class, quality of life, and the distance walked in six minutes.	CRT-D improves quality of life, functional status, and exercise capacity
COMPANION [12]	2004	1520	≤35%	≥120 ms	III-IV	Death from any cause or hospitalization for any cause	CRT-P and CRT-D reduces all cause death and hospitalization
CARE-HF [13]	2005	813	≤35%	≥120 ms	III-IV	Death from any cause, cardiovascular hospitalizations	CRT reduces mortality and heart failure hospitalizations
REVERSE [14]	2008	610	≤40%	≥120 ms	I-II	HF clinical composite response	CRT-P delays time-to-first HF hospitalization and improves in LV end-systolic volume index
MADIT-CRT [15]	2009	1820	≤30%	≥130 ms	I-II	Death from any cause or non-fatal heart failure events	CRT-D reduces heart failure events and all-cause mortality
RAFT [17]	2010	1798	≤30%	≥120 ms	II-III	Death from any cause, heart failure hospitalizations	CRT-D reduces mortality and heart failure hospitalizations
BLOCK-HF [16]	2013	691	≤50%	≥150 ms	I-II	Death, heart failure-related urgent care visits	CRT-P improves clinical outcomes in patients with AV block

Table 1.
A summary of core clinical trials that shaped the current guidelines and selection criteria of CRT [7].

DOI: http://dx.doi.org/10.5772/intechopen.1004423

Recommendation class	Recommendation
Class IA	Patients with LVEF ≤35%, sinus rhythm, LBBB with QRS duration ≥150 ms and NYHA class II-IV on Guideline Directed Medical Therapy (GDMT), CRT with BiV pacing improves symptoms and reduce morbidity and mortality.
Class IIA	Patiens with LVEF ≤35%, sinus rhythm, LBBB with QRS duration ≥150 ms, and NYHA class I symptoms on GDMT, CPP with HBP with LBBB correction or LBBAP is reasonable if effective CRT cannot be achieved with BiV pacing based on anatomical or functional.
Class IIB	In patients with LVEF ≤30%, sinus rhythm, LBBB, QRS duration ≥150 ms, and NYHA class I symptoms on GDMT, CRT with BiV pacing may be considered to reduce the risk of worsening HF and potentially improve LV remodeling.
Class IIB	In patients with LVEF 36–50%, sinus rhythm, LBBB with QRS duration ≥150 ms, and NYHA class II-IV symptoms on GDMT, CPP maybe considered to maintain or improve LVEF
Class IIB	In patients with LVEF <35%, sinus rhythm, LBBB with QRS duration ≥150 ms, and NYHA class II-IV symptoms on GDMT, CSP with HBP or LBBAP may be considered as an alternative to CRT with BIV pacing.

Table 2.
A summary of the 2023 HRS/APHRS/LAHRS guideline on CPP guidelines [1].

4. Indications

This cumulative evidence supporting CRT use in patients with moderate to severe HF and interventricular conduction delay shaped the current guidelines and recommendations. The 2023 HRS/APHRS/LAHRS guideline on CPP support the following (**Table 2**) [1].

5. Patient selection and CRT response

These core CRT clinical trials assessed response on several clinical and echocardiographic parameters. Clinical responses evaluated included NYHA class, improvement in quality of life, increase in peak oxygen consumption, and reduced HF hospitalization and mortality. Echocardiographic responses included >5% absolute increase in LVEF or the absence of worsening in LVEF, reduction in LV size, increase in LV stroke volume, and decrease in mitral regurgitation. Based on these selection criteria, 60–70% of CRT recipients will be responders [1].

Reverse remodeling following CRT has been linked to LBBB, QRS duration (>150 ms), nonischemic etiology, and female sex [18]. Below we discuss the most important predictive factors of CRT response:

5.1 QRS duration and morphology

CRT is effective in patients with QRS duration of >120 to 130 ms. Conversely, individuals with a QRS duration <120 ms are not likely to benefit from CRT based on randomized studies which showed no improvement in peak oxygen consumption or reverse remodeling on the echocardiogram, therefore, CRT is not indicated for this population [19–21]. A comprehensive meta-analysis utilized patient-level data from key

CRT trials, including MIRACLE, MIRACLE-ICD, MIRACLE-ICD II, REVERSE, RAFT, BLOCK-HF, COMPANION, and MADIT-CRT. This meta-analysis aimed to evaluate the benefits of CRT based on QRS morphology LBBB (n = 4549); RBBB, (n = 691); and non-specific intraventricular conduction delay NSIVCD, (n = 1024) and duration (with a 150-ms partition). The primary endpoint focused on the time to heart failure hospitalization (HFH) or death, while a secondary endpoint considered the time to all-cause death. This meta-analysis showed no advantage of CRT in patients with RBBB or NSIVCD [22].

5.2 Cardiomyopathy type (ischemic versus non-ischemic)

In the Cardiac Resynchronization – Heart Failure (CARE-HF) study, CRT resulted in comparable reductions in all-cause mortality for individuals with both ischemic and non-ischemic cardiomyopathy [23]. However, several studies showed that CRT is more effective in patients with non-ischemic cardiomyopathy compared to ischemic cardiomyopathy. CRT in non-ischemic cardiomyopathy resulted in a more substantial increase in LVEF and a greater reduction in NYHA functional class compared to those with ischemic cardiomyopathy [24]. Furthermore, upon conducting sub-analyses of various prospective randomized studies, including MIRACLE (Multicenter InSync Randomized Clinical Evaluation), CARE-HF and, REVERSE (Resynchronization reVErses Remodeling in Systolic left ventricular dysfunction) [20], and MADIT-CRT it was consistently affirmed that more favorable reverse remodeling occurred in cases of non-ischemic cardiomyopathy compared to ischemic cardiomyopathy [25].

5.3 Atrial fibrillation

Frequent atrial arrythmias including atrial fibrillation (AF), and frequent premature ventricular complexes diminish BiV pacing percentage and therefore the CRT effectiveness. Conversely, achieving a high percentage of BiV pacing in observational studies has shown a potential link between CRT and a decreased burden of AF [26]. Regardless, for CRT to be useful, adequate rate control must be present. Achieving a high percentage of BiV pacing proved unsuccessful in approximately two-thirds of the 8686 patients diagnosed with persistent or permanent AF due to medically refractory rapid ventricular rates [27]. Notably, the subgroup with less well controlled rates experienced an elevated risk of mortality. It is important to consider a more aggressive approach to rate control and increased effective BiV pacing in individuals with AF to optimize the advantages of CRT. In fact, in patients with permanent AF in whom primary AF ablation is not possible, many will benefit from AV node ablation and CRT. Specifically, those with heart failure [28]. In the PAVE trial, a group of 184 individuals diagnosed with permanent atrial AF, of which 83% had NYHA class II or III HF, underwent AV node ablation as a treatment for medically refractory rapid ventricular rates. These participants were then randomly allocated to either a standard RV pacing system or CRT pacing system. After a six-month follow-up period, CRT led to significantly greater enhancements in the six-minute walking distance above baseline (31% vs. 24%, $P = 0.04$), peak oxygen consumption during exercise, and exercise duration when compared to standard RV pacing [29].

5.4 LV SCAR

LV scar is detected in as many as 40% of individuals eligible for CRT, and its presence is indicative of an anticipated suboptimal response. Absence of scar in LV and RV pacing regions is associated with 81% CRT response rate compared to when the scar occupies RV pacing region (55% CRT response rate), LV pacing region (25% CRT response rate), and both pacing regions (0% CRT response rate) [30].

6. Pacing considerations in patients with preserved LVEF

Selecting appropriate pacemaker type in patients with bradyarrhythmia and preserved LVEF needs careful consideration. Available choices are RV pacing and CPP (CSP or CRT). Several factors should be considered such as AF, AV conduction and patient's age and comorbidities. Taking these factors into account, both RV pacing and CPP are reasonable options in carefully selected patients.

In PACE, an older study, 177 patients with bradycardia and EF ≥ 45% at baseline were examined for effect if CRT vs. RV only pacing. The EF was better preserved in CRT as compared to those with RV only pacing. In the CRT group, 20.2% dropped their EF ≥5% at 2 year as compared to 62.5% of those in the RV group ($p < 0.001$)[29]. However, no differences were seen in secondary endpoints such as 6-minute walk. Mortality was low in both groups. Thus, mortality benefit was not proven. It is notable that the baseline EF of 45% would by more current standards be regarded as mid-range for heart failure [31]. Similarly, the PREVENT-HF trial, a randomized study involving 108 patients with an initial mean normal LVEF (55% in the RV pacing group and 57% in the CRT group), did not demonstrate a clear advantage of biventricular (BiV) pacing compared to right ventricular pacing (RVP) based on primary and secondary echo parameters of outcome (primary-LV diastolic volume, secondary LV systolic volume, EF and MR). Importantly, while no significant harm was observed with BiV pacing, it is noteworthy that the introduction of an additional left ventricular (LV) lead during the procedure was linked to an extended duration of the procedure and an increased occurrence of procedure-related complications [32].

Based on these data, it is reasonable to perform RV only pacing in patients with preserved EF, particularly in those in whom a low percentage of RV pacing is anticipated. In addition, patients who develop depressed EF because of RV only pacing should be considered for upgrade to CRT [33, 34]. However, it is a class IIb in the HRS/APHRS/LAHRS guidelines to select CPP to reduce the risk of pacemaker-induced cardiomyopathy [1].

7. Procedural considerations and follow up

7.1 Preprocedural evaluation

Preprocedural evaluation includes but is not limited to history and physical exam to evaluate candidacy and severity of HF symptoms, EKG to assess QRS duration and morphology, echocardiogram to evaluate LVEF [35–37]. Rarely, Cardiac MRI (CMR) and nuclear imaging can be used to evaluate LVEF, ischemia and scar.

7.2 CRT implant

Several factors are taken into consideration that can be barriers when performing a CRT implant: engaging the CS, finding optimal branches, and determining the best pacing strategies to maximize CRT. Current guidelines recommend "a quadripolar LV lead to assist with lead stability, lower capture thresholds, avoid phrenic nerve pacing and decrease need for lead repositioning (Class 1)", making lead positioning one of the most important factors to consider when performing CRT device implantation. Compared to bipolar leads, quadripolar leads require less fluoroscopy, allow for better distal vein positioning, and facilitate lower pacing thresholds and impedances [38]. Given that pacing vectors can be switched between the different poles, phrenic nerve stimulation can be avoided. Thus, the best hemodynamic response is usually achieved by placing the electrode around the area with the latest LV activation that provides adequate threshold without phrenic nerve stimulation.

Moreover, there are several means of optimization of CRT therapy. In a small study [39], the best hemodynamic response was achieved with the narrowest QRS duration by optimization of the interventricular delay. Additional improvement in reverse remodeling can be achieved by optimizing the AV delay and finding the best fusion-optimized QRS duration during LV pacing [40]. Currently, device manufacturers have different algorithms to enhance QRS duration automatically to provide an individual approach to each patient. For example, certain Medtronic CRT device models use AdaptivCRT™ algorithm which enhances physiological and dynamic pacing by assessing intrinsic conduction to determine appropriate AV interval duration, based on the AV interval, the device decides on Adaptive LV vs. BiV pacing. As a result, the device will continuously optimize the AV and VV delay and optimize pacing configuration [41]. Several studies have shown non-inferiority of this method compared to echocardiographic optimization which is time consuming and rarely performed clinically.

Anatomic lead positioning is also fundamental and plays an important role in the success of a CRT. Apical LV pacing has shown lower event-free survival and LV reverse remodeling compared to basal and midventricular LV lead positions [42]. Additionally, placement of LV leads in areas of electrical delay can confer a greater benefit [43]. QLV (time from the onset of QRS on the ECG to local activation at the site of the LV lead) > 95 ms or > 50% total QRS duration favor optimal response with CRT.

When CS lead placement is unattainable, surgical epicardial LV lead pacing is a reasonable alternative.

7.3 Complications

The risks of complications should be weighed when deciding to implant a CRT device. In those with life expectancy <1, shared decision-making is required to consider the potential improvement in quality of life compared to the risk of procedural complications. CRT-D is not indicated for these patients, whereas CRT-P may be considered.

The complications related to a CRT are those inherent to a pacemaker and ICD with the addition of those related to an LV lead placement. These complications include coronary vein dissection or perforation. Additionally, other complications include the risk of pneumothorax, lead dislodgement, infection and/or hematoma, perforation, tamponade, cardiac arrest, and sustained ventricular tachyarrhythmia.

7.4 Follow up

A multidisciplinary team is required for follow up of patients with implanted CRT devices. This includes advanced heart failure and electrophysiologists, both to assess and optimize GDMT and assess periodically LV lead capture. This is best accomplished in a specialized device clinic [44]. Patients who do not appear to have benefited from CRT need careful evaluation to correct potentially reversible factors, such as inadequate BiV pacing percentage (due to a high burden of ectopy or AF), or suboptimal lead placement position. A chest X-ray can be useful to assess LV lead position. A 12-lead ECG is useful to confirm LV capture and facilitate optimization of LV pacing configurations. An echocardiogram should be repeated within 3–12 months after implant. Ablation or pharmacological suppression of PVCs or atrial fibrillation might be required to promote enhanced BiV pacing.

7.5 Alternatives to CRT

LV lead placement is not possible in up to 10% of patients planned for CRT with BiV pacing due to anatomical/technical reasons, functional issues (high thresholds, diaphragmatic stimulation), and intrinsic ECG considerations. Criteria for optimal lead placement continue to evolve and failure of lead placement at initial implantation has not been standardized. Hence, the decision to abandon the initial approach and crossover to another conduction system pacing (HBP or LBBAP) varies among the operators. Current guidelines recommend crossover from CRT with BiV pacing via CS to CSP with HBP or LBBAP when the CS LV lead placement is unsuccessful or suboptimal (class 2a). Crossover to epicardial LV lead placement is currently a class 2b indication.

We are not fully addressing CSP in this chapter, but briefly note that there is compelling data to support the use of CSP, either as a "fallback" when CRT is not feasible. Or in some cases as a preferred first line means to achieve resynchronization.

7.6 Response to CRT

The response to CRT in heart failure patients is variable. Some may experience improvement in objective (LVEF, NYHA class) and/or subjective parameters and in some others, CRT might manifest as a slowing of the natural progression of HF [45]. In all these patients, continuation of CRT should be sought at the time of battery replacement as some studies have shown worse outcomes when CRT was deactivated in people with improved LVEF [46]. Those who do not respond to CRT as expected are labeled as "nonresponders". However, this definition does not consider the natural history of the disease and the fact that CRT can stabilize HF progression. Nevertheless, these patients should have medication optimization, evaluation of lead position, device reprogramming to optimize and look for a favorable response.

8. Future directions and innovation

8.1 Leadless CRT

Leadless pacemaker implantation is growing due to the high success rate and low complication rate [47]. Single and dual chamber leadless pacemaker eliminates leads and generator-related complications such as lead fracture or dislodgement, and pocket infection or procedural complications such as pneumothorax and coronary sinus perforation [48]. Leadless CRT efficacy and safety remains under investigation, however, similar to single and dual chamber leadless pacemakers, leadless CRT will eliminate lead and some procedural complications compared to conventional CRT.

The SOLVE-CRT study, presented at Heart Rhythm 2023 scientific meeting, introduced the WiSE® CRT System, a potential endocardial LV pacing as an alternative to conventional CRT. The study included CRT non-responders, untreated cases with lead failures, and those undergoing high-risk upgrades. Results showed 80.9% freedom from Type I complications (device and procedure-related) and a significant 16.4% improvement in Left Ventricular End Systolic Volume [49]. Although a large sample randomized double blinded clinical trials are needed to determine the efficacy and safety of leadless CRT, these positive findings will help customize CRT in HF patients.

8.2 Use of advanced cardiac imaging to optimize response and patient selection

QRS duration as the sole measurement of ventricular dyssyncrhony is not ideal. This is evidenced by the 30% CRT nonresponse rate. Nonresponders may include a subset with wide QRS but no actual mechanical dyssyncrhony. This inspired researchers to evaluate other methods to predict CRT responsiveness and optimize patient selection. Initially, echocardiogram offered a non-electrical assessment of mechanical dyssnchrony using several parameters such as M-mode, color tissue Doppler (TD) M-mode, longitudinal TD velocity, pulsed TD, additional measures such as strain and strain rate imaging and 3-D echocardiography [50]. However, the multicentric Predictors of Response to CRT (PROSPECT) study showed variable ability of echocardiographic parameters to predict CRT response, sensitivity (ranging from 6–74%) and specificity (ranging from 35–91%) [51]. Similarly, echocardiographic characterization of dyssynchrony in patients with QRS <130 ms in the Cardiac-Resynchronization Therapy in Heart Failure with a Narrow QRS Complex trial failed to improve outcomes in the study population prompting halting the study due to safety concerns [52]. As a result, failure of echocardiographic assessment of mechanical dyssyncrhony opened the avenue for alternative imaging approach.

Various MRI-based methods and indices have been established to improve CRT patient selection and optimize pacing algorithm. CMR may be useful to predict the CRT responsiveness and improve patient selection and predict long term outcomes. Techniques such as cine myocardial tagging, harmonic phase analysis, and strain-encoded MRI offer a more comprehensive evaluation of ventricular dyssyncrhony [53, 54]. Taylor AJ et al. demonstrated the utility of multisequential CMR in predicting CRT response. Mechanical dyssyncrhony identified as ≥65 ms delay between septal and posterolateral wall contraction on cine imaging in combination with lack of transmural scarring of the anteroseptal or posterolateral wall on delayed contrast-enhanced imaging were labeled as CRT-responders. The sensitivity of CMR-predicted CRT clinical response was 90%, with a specificity of 59%. Additionally, transplant-free survival post-CRT was observed in 88% in CMR-predicted CRT responders vs. 58% in CMR-predicted non-responders [55].

Myocardial tagging is a CMR technique that uses temporary tags applied to the myocardium to monitor myocardial deformation and motion throughout the cardiac cycle. Bilchick KC et al. using a circumferential mechanical dyssynchrony index (Circumferential Uniformity Ratio Estimate or CURE), a value derived from myocardial tagging, was able to predict clinical response in CRT HF group with 90% accurate rate. The addition of scar imaging improved the accuracy rate to 95%. This study demonstrates the use of myocardial tagging-CURE combined with scar imaging predicts clinical responsiveness after CRT with 95% accuracy rate [56]. Chalil S et al. evaluated the Cardiovascular Magnetic Resonance-Tissue Synchronization Index (CMR-TSI) ability to independently predict major cardiovascular events in CRT patients. CMR-TSI ≥110 ms was associated with worse outcomes including death or unplanned HF hospitalization [57].

8.3 Artificial intelligence

Artificial Intelligence (AI) and Machine Learning (ML) is at the forefront of cardiovascular medicine. CRT-respondent patient selection remains challenging. AI and ML may be able to provide better classification and characterization of heart failure patients with ventricular dyssyncrhony. Cikes M et al. applied unsupervised machine learning algorithm on 1106 HF patients from the MADIT-CRT dataset utilizing echocardiographic and clinical data to phenotype heart failure patients to identify CRT respondents. This algorithm, groups patients with similarities in clinical parameters, LV volume, and deformation traces at baseline. Four phenogroups were identified, two of these groups had higher clinical characteristics predictive of CRT response [58]. Similarly, Feeny AK et al. used a ML algorithm incorporating 9 variables including QRS morphology, QRS duration, New York Heart Association classification, left ventricular ejection fraction, end-diastolic diameter, sex, ischemic cardiomyopathy, atrial fibrillation, and epicardial left ventricular lead. This model was superior to guidelines in predicting CRT responsiveness and survival [59]. AI and ML serve as an essential building block in predicting CRT responsiveness and outcomes.

9. Conclusion

Decades of research has led to impressive gains in knowledge of the interplay between cardiac conduction abnormalities, symptoms, morbidity and mortality. Impressive strides have been made at correcting electromechanical dyssynchrony. The evidence supporting CRT benefits in selected patients with symptomatic HFrEF and dyssyncrhony is overwhelming. CRT therapy improves quality of life and reduces mortality. When CRT is not feasible, CSP provides a good alternative. Future directions at better patient selection and improved technology hold great promise.

Conflict of interest

The authors declare no conflict of interest.

Author details

Malik Ghawanmeh, Dorys Chavez*, Luis Cerna Urrutia and Cynthia M. Tracy
George Washington University School of Medicine and Health Sciences,
Washington, DC, United States

*Address all correspondence to: dorys.arlene@gmail.com

References

[1] Chung MK, Patton KK, Lau CP, et al. 2023 HRS/APHRS/LAHRS guideline on cardiac physiologic pacing for the avoidance and mitigation of heart failure. Heart Rhythm. 2023;**20**:e17-e91

[2] Soman P, Malhotra S. Left bundle branch block and cardiac resynchronization therapy: Effector or bystander? Circulation. Cardiovascular Imaging. Nov 2022;**15**(11):1-3. DOI: 10.1161/circimaging.122.014849

[3] Eriksson J, Zajac J, Alehagen U, Bolger AF, Ebbers T, Carlhäll C-J. Left ventricular hemodynamic forces as a marker of mechanical dyssynchrony in heart failure patients with left bundle branch block. Scientific Reports. 7 Jun 2017;**7**(1):1-4. DOI: 10.1038/s41598-017-03089-x

[4] Tan NY, Witt CM, Oh JK, Cha Y-M. Left bundle branch block. Circulation: Arrhythmia and Electrophysiology. Apr 2020;**13**(4):1-11. DOI: 10.1161/circep.119.008239

[5] Sciarra L, Golia P, Palamà Z, Scarà A, De Ruvo E, Borrelli A, et al. Patients with left bundle branch block and left axis deviation show a specific left ventricular asynchrony pattern: Implications for left ventricular lead placement during CRT implantation. Journal of Electrocardiology. 2018;**51**(2):175-181. DOI: 10.1016/j.jelectrocard.2017.10.006

[6] Leclercq C, Gras D, Le Helloco A, et al. Hemodynamic importance of preserving the normal sequence of ventricular activation in permanent cardiac pacing. American Heart Journal. 1995;**129**:1133

[7] Leyva F, Nisam S, Auricchio A. 20 years of cardiac resynchronization therapy. Journal of the American College of Cardiology. 2014;**64**:1047-1058

[8] Cazeau S, Leclercq C, Lavergne T, et al. Effects of multisite biventricular pacing in patients with heart failure and intraventricular conduction delay. The New England Journal of Medicine. 2001;**344**:873-880

[9] Auricchio A, Stellbrink C, Sack S, et al. Long-term clinical effect of hemodynamically optimized cardiac resynchronization therapy in patients with heart failure and ventricular conduction delay. Journal of the American College of Cardiology. 2002;**39**:2026-2033

[10] Abraham WT, Fisher WG, Smith AL, et al. Cardiac resynchronization in chronic heart failure. The New England Journal of Medicine. 2002;**346**:1845-1853

[11] Young JB, Abraham WT, Smith AL, et al. Combined cardiac resynchronization and implantable cardioversion defibrillation in advanced chronic heart failure: The MIRACLE ICD Trial. JAMA. 2003;**289**:2685-2694

[12] Bristow MR, Saxon LA, Boehmer J, et al. Cardiac-resynchronization therapy with or without an implantable defibrillator in advanced chronic heart failure. The New England Journal of Medicine. 2004;**350**:2140-2150

[13] Cleland JG, Daubert JC, Erdmann E, et al. The effect of cardiac resynchronization on morbidity and mortality in heart failure. The New England Journal of Medicine. 2005;**352**:1539-1549

[14] Linde C, Abraham WT, Gold MR, St John Sutton M, Ghio S, Daubert C.

Randomized trial of cardiac resynchronization in mildly symptomatic heart failure patients and in asymptomatic patients with left ventricular dysfunction and previous heart failure symptoms. Journal of the American College of Cardiology. 2008;**52**:1834-1843

[15] Moss AJ, Hall WJ, Cannom DS, et al. Cardiac-resynchronization therapy for the prevention of heart-failure events. The New England Journal of Medicine. 2009;**361**:1329-1338

[16] Curtis AB, Worley SJ, Adamson PB, et al. Biventricular pacing for atrioventricular block and systolic dysfunction. The New England Journal of Medicine. 2013;**368**:1585-1593

[17] Tang AS, Wells GA, Talajic M, et al. and for the resynchronization-defibrillation for ambulatory heart failure trial investigators : "Cardiac-resynchronization therapy for mild-to-moderate heart failure". The New England Journal of Medicine. 2010;**363**:2385

[18] Goldenberg I, Moss AJ, Hall WJ, Foster E, Goldberger JJ, Santucci P, et al. Predictors of response to cardiac resynchronization therapy in the Multicenter automatic defibrillator implantation trial with cardiac resynchronization therapy (MADIT-CRT). Circulation. 2011;**124**:1527-1536

[19] Poole JE, Singh JP, Birgersdotter-Green U. QRS duration or QRS morphology. Journal of the American College of Cardiology. 2016;**67**(9):1104-1117. DOI: 10.1016/j.jacc.2015.12.039

[20] John Sutton M, Ghio S, Plappert T, Tavazzi L, Scelsi L, Daubert C, et al. Cardiac resynchronization induces major structural and functional reverse remodeling in patients with New York Heart Association class I/II heart failure. Circulation. 2009;**120**(19):1858-1865. DOI: 10.1161/circulationaha.108.818724

[21] Beshai JF, Grimm RA, Nagueh SF, Baker JH, Beau SL, Greenberg SM, et al. Cardiac-resynchronization therapy in heart failure with narrow QRS complexes. New England Journal of Medicine. 2007;**357**(24):2461-2471. DOI: 10.1056/nejmoa0706695

[22] Friedman DJ, Al-Khatib SM, Dalgaard F, Fudim M, Abraham WT, Cleland JGF, et al. Cardiac resynchronization therapy improves outcomes in patients with intraventricular conduction delay but not right bundle branch block: A patient-level metaanalysis of randomized controlled trials. Circulation. 7 Mar 2023;**147**(10):812-823. DOI: 10.1161/circulationaha.122.062124

[23] WikstromG, Blomstrom-LundqvistC, Andren B, Lonnerholm S, Blomstrom P, Freemantle N, et al. The effects of aetiology on outcome in patients treated with cardiac resynchronization therapy in the care-HF trial. European Heart Journal. 2008;**30**(7):782-788. DOI: 10.1093/eurheartj/ehn577

[24] Gasparini M, Mantica M, Galimberti P, Genovese L, Pini D, Faletra F, et al. Is the outcome of cardiac resynchronization therapy related to the underlying etiology? Pacing and Clinical Electrophysiology. 2003;**26**(1):175-180. DOI: 10.1046/j.1460-9592.2003.00011.x

[25] Barsheshet A, Goldenberg I, Moss AJ, Eldar M, Huang DT, McNitt S, et al. Response to preventive cardiac resynchronization therapy in patients with ischaemic and nonischaemic cardiomyopathy in madit-CRT. European Heart Journal. 2010;**32**(13):1622-1630. DOI: 10.1093/eurheartj/ehq407

[26] Fung JW-H, Yu C-M, Chan JY-S, Chan HC-K, Yip GW-K, Zhang Q, et al. Effects of cardiac resynchronization therapy on incidence of atrial fibrillation in patients with poor left ventricular systolic function. The American Journal of Cardiology. 2005;**96**(5):728-731. DOI: 10.1016/j.amjcard.2005.04.053

[27] Jacobsson J, Reitan C, Carlson J, Borgquist R, Platonov PG. Atrial fibrillation incidence and impact of biventricular pacing on long-term outcome in patients with heart failure treated with cardiac resynchronization therapy. BMC Cardiovascular Disorders. 13 Aug 2019;**195**(1):1-9. DOI: 10.1186/s12872-019-1169-1

[28] Gasparini M, Regoli F, Galimberti P, Ceriotti C, Cappelleri A. Cardiac resynchronization therapy in heart failure patients with atrial fibrillation. Europace. 2009;**11**(Supplement 5):v82-v86. DOI: 10.1093/europace/eup273

[29] Doshi RN, Daoud EG, Fellows C, Turk K, Duran A, Hamdan MH, et al. Left ventricular-based cardiac stimulation post AV nodal ablation evaluation (the PAVE study). Journal of Cardiovascular Electrophysiology. 2005;**16**(11):1160-1165. DOI: 10.1111/j.1540-8167.2005.50062.x

[30] Wong JA, Yee R, Stirrat J, Scholl D, Krahn AD, Gula LJ, et al. Influence of pacing site characteristics on response to cardiac resynchronization therapy. Circulation. Cardiovascular Imaging. 2013;**6**(4):542-550. DOI: 10.1161/circimaging.111.000146

[31] Habel N, Infeld M, Bernknopf J, Meyer M, Lustgarten D. Rationale and design of the pace HFPEF trial: Physiologic accelerated pacing as a holistic treatment of heart failure with preserved ejection fraction. Heart Rhythm O2. 2024;**5**(1):41-49. DOI: 10.1016/j.hroo.2023.12.001

[32] Heidenreich PA, Bozkurt B, Aguilar D, Allen LA, Byun JJ, Colvin MM, et al. AHA/ACC/HFSA guideline for the management of heart failure. Journal of the American College of Cardiology. 2022;**79**(17):895-1032. DOI: 10.1016/j.jacc.2021.12.012

[33] Stockburger M, Gómez-Doblas JJ, Lamas G, Alzueta J, Fernández-Lozano I, Cobo E, et al. Preventing ventricular dysfunction in pacemaker patients without advanced heart failure: Results from a multicentre international randomized trial (prevent-hf). European Journal of Heart Failure. 2011;**13**(6):633-641. DOI: 10.1093/eurjhf/hfr041

[34] Shetty AK, Rinaldi CA. Cardiac resynchronization therapy upgrade. Circulation: Arrhythmia and Electrophysiology. 2017;**10**(2):004956. DOI: 10.1161/circep.117.004956

[35] Slotwiner DJ, Raitt MH, Del-Carpio Munoz F, Mulpuru SK, Nasser N, Peterson PN. Impact of physiologic pacing versus right ventricular pacing among patients with left ventricular ejection fraction greater than 35%: A systematic review for the 2018 ACC/AHA/HRS guideline on the evaluation and management of patients with bradycardia and cardiac conduction delay. Heart Rhythm. 2019;**16**(9):e280-e298. DOI: 10.1016/j.hrthm.2018.10.035

[36] Sipahi I, Chou JC, Hyden M, Rowland DY, Simon DI, Fang JC. Effect of QRS morphology on clinical event reduction with cardiac resynchronization therapy: Meta-analysis of randomized controlled trials. American Heart Journal. 2012;**163**:260-267.e3

[37] Birnie DH, Ha A, Higginson L, Sidhu K, Green M, Philippon F, et al. Impact of QRS morphology and duration on outcomes after cardiac

resynchronization therapy. Circulation. Heart Failure. 2013;**6**:1190-1198

[38] Linde C, Abraham WT, Gold MR, John Sutton M, Ghio S, Daubert C. Randomized trial of cardiac resynchronization in mildly symptomatic heart failure patients and in asymptomatic patients with left ventricular dysfunction and previous heart failure symptoms. Journal of the American College of Cardiology. 2008;**52**:1834-1843

[39] Glikson M, Nielsen JC, Kronborg MB, Michowitz Y, Auricchio A, Barbash IM, et al. 2021 ESC guidelines on cardiac pacing and cardiac resynchronization therapy: Developed by the task force on cardiac pacing and cardiac resynchronization therapy of the European Society of Cardiology (ESC) with the special contribution of the European Heart Rhythm Association (EHRA). European Heart Journal. 2021;**42**:3427-3520

[40] Tamborero D, Mont L, Sitges M, Silva E, Berruezo A, Vidal B, et al. Optimization of the interventricular delay in cardiac resynchronization therapy using the QRS width. The American Journal of Cardiology. 2009;**104**:1407-1412

[41] Trucco E, Tolosana JM, Arbelo E, Doltra A, Castel M, Benito E, et al. Improvement of reverse Remodeling using electrocardiogram fusion-optimized intervals in cardiac resynchronization therapy: A randomized study. JACC Clinical Electrophysiology. 2018;**4**:181-189

[42] Birnie D, Hudnall H, Lemke B, et al. Continuous optimization of cardiac resynchronization therapy reduces atrial fibrillation in heart failure patients: Results of the adaptive cardiac resynchronization therapy trial. Heart Rhythm. 2017;**14**:1820-1825

[43] Thébault C, Donal E, Meunier C, Gervais R, Gerritse B, Gold MR, et al. Sites of left and right ventricular lead implantation and response to cardiac resynchronization therapy observations from the REVERSE trial. European Heart Journal. 2012;**33**:2662-2671

[44] Parreira L, Tsyganov A, Artyukhina E, Vernooy K, Tondo C, Adragao P, et al. Non-invasive three-dimensional electrical activation mapping to predict cardiac resynchronization therapy response: Site of latest left ventricular activation relative to pacing site. EP Europace. 2023;**25**:1458-1466

[45] Altman RK, Parks KA, Schlett CL, Orencole M, Park M-Y, Truong QA, et al. Multidisciplinary care of patients receiving cardiac resynchronization therapy is associated with improved clinical outcomes. European Heart Journal. 2012;**33**:2181-2188

[46] Gold MR, Rickard J, Daubert JC, Zimmerman P, Linde C. Redefining the classifications of response to cardiac resynchronization therapy: Results from the REVERSE study. JACC: Clinical Electrophysiology. 2021;**7**:871-880

[47] Cay S, Ozeke O, Ozcan F, Aras D, Topaloglu S. Mid-term clinical and echocardiographic evaluation of super responders with and without pacing: The preliminary results of a prospective, randomized, single-Centre study. EP Europace. 2015;**18**:842-850

[48] Roberts PR, Clementy N, Al Samadi F, et al. A leadless pacemaker in the real-world setting: The Micra Transcatheter pacing system post-approval registry. Heart Rhythm. 2017;**14**:1375-1379

[49] van Rees JB, de Bie MK, Thijssen J, Borleffs CJ, Schalij MJ, van Erven L. Implantation-related complications of

implantable cardioverter-defibrillators and cardiac resynchronization therapy devices: A systematic review of randomized clinical trials. Journal of the American College of Cardiology. 2011;**58**:995-1000

[50] Okabe T, Hummel JD, Bank AJ, et al. Leadless left ventricular stimulation with WiSE-CRT system – initial experience and results from phase I of SOLVE-CRT Study (nonrandomized, roll-in phase). Heart Rhythm. 2022;**19**:22-29

[51] Gorcsan J, Abraham T, Agler DA, et al. Echocardiography for cardiac resynchronization therapy: recommendations for performance and reporting--a report from the American Society of Echocardiography Dyssynchrony Writing Group endorsed by the Heart Rhythm Society. Journal of the American Society of Echocardiography. 2008;**21**:191-213

[52] Chung ES, Leon AR, Tavazzi L, et al. Results of the predictors of response to CRT (PROSPECT) trial. Circulation. 2008;**117**:2608-2616

[53] Ruschitzka F, Abraham WT, Singh JP, et al. Cardiac-resynchronization therapy in heart failure with a narrow QRS complex. The New England Journal of Medicine. 2013;**369**:1395-1405

[54] Lardo AC, Abraham TP, Kass DA. Magnetic resonance imaging assessment of ventricular dyssynchrony: Current and emerging concepts. Journal of the American College of Cardiology. 2005;**46**:2223-2228

[55] Taylor AJ, Elsik M, Broughton A, et al. Combined dyssynchrony and scar imaging with cardiac magnetic resonance imaging predicts clinical response and long-term prognosis following cardiac resynchronization therapy. Europace. 2010;**12**:708-713

[56] Bilchick KC, Dimaano V, Wu KC, et al. Cardiac magnetic resonance assessment of dyssynchrony and myocardial scar predicts function class improvement following cardiac resynchronization therapy. JACC: Cardiovascular Imaging. 2008;**1**:561-568

[57] Chalil S, Stegemann B, Muhyaldeen S, et al. Intraventricular dyssynchrony predicts mortality and morbidity after cardiac resynchronization therapy: A study using cardiovascular magnetic resonance tissue synchronization imaging. Journal of the American College of Cardiology. 2007;**50**:243-252

[58] Cikes M, Sanchez-Martinez S, Claggett B, et al. Machine learning-based phenogrouping in heart failure to identify responders to cardiac resynchronization therapy. European Journal of Heart Failure. 2019;**21**:74-85

[59] Feeny AK, Rickard J, Patel D, et al. Machine learning prediction of response to cardiac resynchronization therapy: Improvement versus current guidelines. Circulation. Arrhythmia and Electrophysiology. 2019;**12**:e007316

Chapter 5

Cardiac Resynchronization Therapy Devices Implantation Technique

Radu Darciuc

Abstract

This chapter describes the most important technical aspects of the cardiac resynchronization therapy device implantation. It includes the technique of anesthesia, venous access, pocket creation, coronary sinus cannulation, left ventricular lead placement, etc. The description of the necessary tools is made to help implanting physicians become familiar with and overcome possible challenges during the procedure. We compare several techniques for every step, underlining their advantages and disadvantages. We mention a list of tip and tricks that will help physicians perform implantations and become more proficient. Numerous figures and images are used to make the explanation of the technique more comprehensive.

Keywords: coronary sinus cannulation, generator pocket, left ventricular lead placement, target vessel, venous access

1. Introduction

In the last decades, cardiac resynchronization therapy (CRT) has become a strategic treatment for patients with advanced heart failure and left bundle branch block (LBBB).

In 1994, Cazeau et al. published their paper about the first successful cases of biventricular pacing in patients with severe congestive heart failure [1], in 1998, Daubert et al. published about transvenous approach via the coronary sinus (CS) tributaries [2] leading to fast development of various techniques and tools for CRT.

Nowadays, CRT device implantation has become a routine technique performed in many specialized centers around the globe. Nevertheless, during the procedure, some challenges and complications may arise. This is why it is important to have proper knowledge and tools.

A lot of information about the technical aspects of the CRT device implantation was gained during years: about choice of anesthesia, venous access, pocket creation, coronary sinus cannulation, left ventricular lead placement, etc.

2. Patient preparation

The success of the CRT device implantation starts with the preparation of the patient. That preoperatory part is very important. Before the procedure, we take into consideration aspects such as:

- Stopping or adjusting anticoagulants

For years, bridging anticoagulation was performed before implantation in patients taking oral anticoagulation. Nowadays, some centers do not even discontinue anticoagulants before the procedure. Other centers act in a case-by-case manner, as was mentioned by AlTurki et al. [3].

The current approach in our center is:

In patients on direct oral anticoagulants, we give the last dose 24–48 hours before the procedure for Rivaroxaban and 12–24 hours for Dabigatran or Apixaban. In patients on Antivitamin K anticoagulants (Warfarin, Acenocoumarol) and international normalized ratio (INR) > 2.5 we stop them 2 days before the procedure. If INR is ~2 we do not stop the anticoagulants.

- The placement of the peripheral venous catheter

The catheter has to be placed on the same side where the device is implanted.

Why is that important? It is important to have the venous catheter at that side in case the venogram of the cephalic, axillary, and subclavian veins will be necessary to guide the puncture.

- Antibiotic prophylaxis

According to the current guidelines [4], it is important to give 2 g intravenous cefazolin (or 3 g in patients over 120 kg), 30–60 minutes before the procedure. In patients with known allergy to cephalosporin, 1 g of vancomycin is administered before the procedure in slow infusion (during 2 hours).

We recommend the use of the Prevention of Arrhythmia Device Infection Trial (PADIT) score to predict the risk of infection [5]. In patients with a PADIT score of ≥5 points, we continue with oral antibiotic therapy for 5–7 days after the procedure.

3. Anesthesia

CRT device implantation is a minor surgical procedure and is performed under local anesthesia.

Usually, local anesthesia with lidocaine is used. Three syringes with 4 ml Lidocaine 2% diluted with 6 ml sodium chloride 0.9% are usually enough to perform the case.

If the patient has an allergy to lidocaine, we could choose another local anesthetic such as bupivacaine or articaine.

Is the sedation necessary? It could be used because it adds comfort for both physician and patient. The sedation is obtained with 1–6 mg midazolam and 25–100 μg fentanyl, or deep sedation with continuous propofol infusion could be performed in unstable patients.

4. Venous access

An important part of the procedure is the venous access. Several different techniques of venous access exist, such as cephalic vein preparation, subclavian vein access, and axillary vein access. Which one to choose?

The cephalic vein is, in many cases, not suitable for implanting all three leads. The subclavian puncture has more risks. This is why our current approach is to use axillary vein puncture. It permits access to the extrathoracic portion of the venous system, leading to decreased risk of pneumothorax formation and avoidance of lead fractures. In our center, we had no pneumothorax complications when the axillary vein was punctured but had some when subclavian vein access was chosen [6].

How to guide the puncture?

Some operators use ultrasound to guide axillary vein puncture, some use anatomical landmarks only, and some use X-ray landmarks to guide the puncture. In our center, we use the X-ray-guided axillary vein puncture technique described by Burri et al. [7]. The target point for the pucture is the confluence of the second and third rib, where the vein is usually located. With fluoroscopy guidance, we advance the needle, pointing toward the head of the patient at a 45–60° angle to the skin surface until the blood is aspirated. To avoid pneumothorax, we take care not to cross the medial border of the first rib.

What if we cannot find the vein? It could happen if the patient is dehydrated, if there is venous spasm, or if there is venous occlusion. What to do in such a case? If the venous access is challenging, it is advisable to perform a venogram. For that is necessary to inject about 10 ml of contrast agent (iohexol 350 mg/ml) diluted with 10 ml 0.9% sodium chloride in the peripheral venous catheter. The contrast agent flows through the venous system and permits us to obtain the image of the cephalic, axillary, and subclavian veins. The venogram is latter used as a reference image to guide the vein puncture.

5. Pocket

We will not describe in detail the location of the incision. There are different approaches, taking into consideration which venous access was chosen and some cosmetic aspects.

In case a CRT device with defibrillator (CRT-D) is implanted, a subpectoral generator implantation has to be taken into consideration. It permits us to obtain better cosmetic results and avoid skin erosion, especially in patients with frailty. In patients with well-developed subcutaneous tissue, a prepectoral pocket could be created.

6. Leads placement

After obtaining the venous access, the peel-away sheath introducer is inserted in the vein, and the lead is advanced into the heart chambers.

Right ventricular (RV) lead is used for pacing, sensing, and, in case of a CRT-D device, for delivery of shocks. Right atrial (RA) lead is used for pacing and sensing. The left ventricular (LV) lead is used for pacing and sensing.

6.1 Which leads to implant first?

The majority of operators perform RV lead placement first. That approach has some specific advantages. We obtain a landmark for CS cannulation with the RV lead curve [8].

It helps us to understand the location of the CS ostium. Another advantage is that we also have the lead in place if an emergency pacing is needed, for example, in case of asystole.

6.2 Where to secure the RV lead?

It could be placed in an apical or septal position. The apical position is more stable but has more risks of cardiac perforation.

6.3 Is RA lead always necessary?

The question about RA lead could gain interest if the patient has permanent atrial fibrillation. Is it necessary to implant the RA lead? Yes, it is necessary. The RA lead has to be implanted even in patients with permanent atrial fibrillation, taking into consideration the possibility of the conversion to sinus rhythm (spontaneous or after delivery of shocks). Also, the RA lead presence is used by arrythmia discrimination algorithms of the device.

6.4 Coronary sinus cannulation

The basic lead for CRT is the LV lead that is placed in the coronary sinus. The LV lead placement is the main part of the procedure, which is sometimes technically difficult and time-consuming.

The most important and challenging step in LV lead placement is CS ostium cannulation.

How to cannulate the CS ostium?

We can use different techniques [9–11]:

- direct cannulation with the CS sheath
- use of the electrophysiology (EP) catheters
- use of the coronarography catheters (AL2, MP catheters).

Every center or physician has his own style, but it could be performed as follows, using several consecutive techniques:

1. Direct cannulation with the CS (**Figure 1**).

   The J-shaped guidewire is gently placed in the RV, and the CS sheath is pushed over the guidewire. We aim to place the tip of the sheath over the tricuspid valve (near the RV lead curve) (**Figure 1B**). Then we pull back the guidewire. After that, we gently rotate counterclockwise and pull back the CS. With that rotation, the tip of the CS sheath usually jumps in the CS ostium. We confirm the engagement by injecting some contrast, and if confirmed, cannulate the CS with the guidewire and thereafter with the CS sheath over the wire.

2. The use of the EP catheters (**Figure 2**).

   To perform that type of cannulation, we insert 6F or 7F deflectable (or non-deflectable) EP catheters inside the CS sheath. The shape of the catheter could

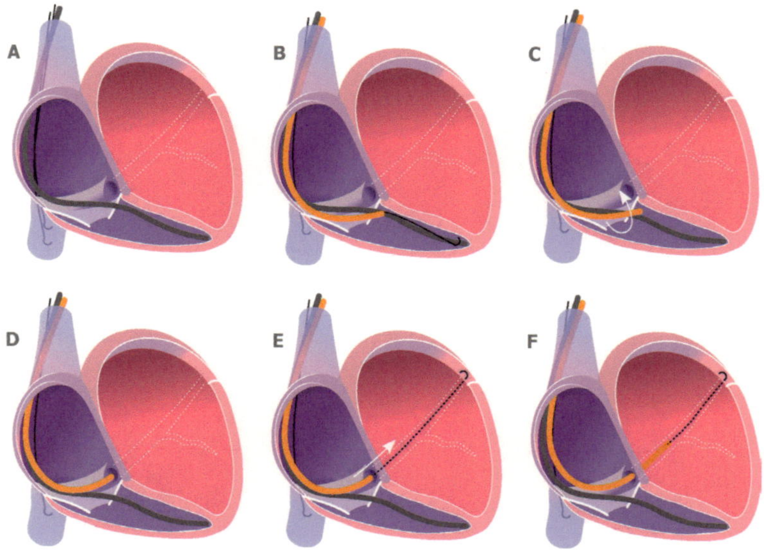

Figure 1.
Coronary sinus cannulation using coronary sinus sheath. A. The right ventricle lead is in place. Two J-shaped guidewires parked in the inferior vena cava. B. One of the guidewires is placed in the right ventricle, and the coronary sinus sheath is pushed over the guidewire on the tricuspid valve. C. The guidewire is pulled back into the coronary sinus sheath, and the sheath is rotated counterclockwise. D. The tip of the sheath at the coronary sinus ostium. E. The J-shaped guidewire is advanced into the coronary sinus. F. The coronary sinus sheath is advanced over the J-shaped guidewire and inserted into the coronary sinus.

be changed adjusting to the CS ostium position. Also, the tip of EP catheter is round. Therefore, the risk of CS dissection is lower. Some operators use not only anatomical landmarks to guide the cannulation but also electrograms obtained from the EP catheter. After cannulating the CS with the EP catheter, we push the CS sheath over the EP catheter inside the CS.

3. Another technique to find the CS ostium in difficult cases is the use of small amount of contrast agent. The operator is gently moving the tip of the CS sheath and injects small amounts of contrast. When the CS ostium is located, it is directly cannulated with the CS sheath or with the J-shaped guidewire.

4. Coronarography with venous phase. When we cannot find the ostium with the techniques mentioned above, we can think about performing coronarography with the venous phase. It allows us to understand the CS anatomy and to use the obtained venogram as a reference image.

5. The telescopic method. In some challenging cases, the operator can use additional catheters inside the main CS sheath. Different types of coronarography catheters such as AL2, AL3, and MP could be used to enter the CS ostium (**Figure 3**).

Sometimes, even when using all the mentioned techniques, we cannot engage the CS ostium. What to do in such a case? We have at least three options: to postpone the procedure for other session, use left bundle branch (LBB) area pacing, or refer to cardiac surgeons for epicardial LV pacing.

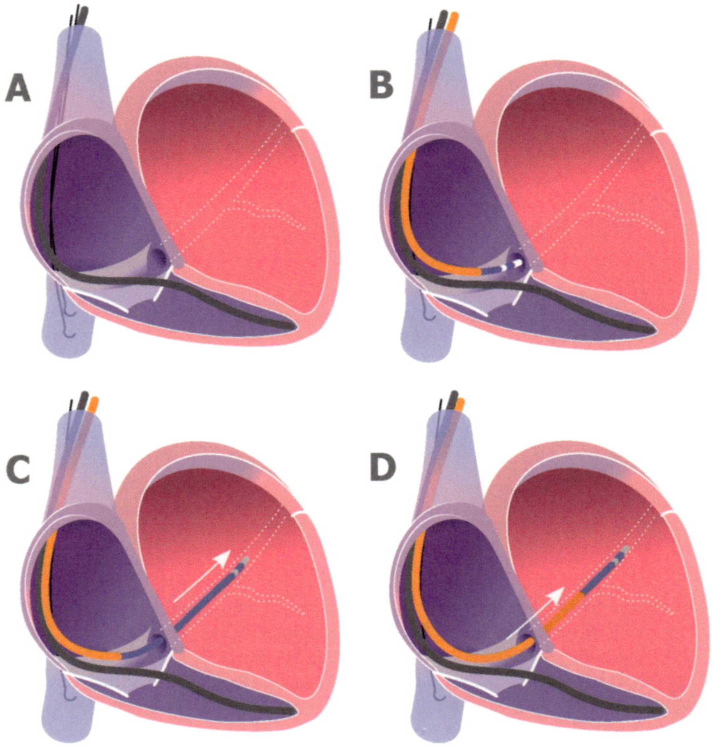

Figure 2.
Coronary sinus cannulation using electrophysiology catheter. A. The right ventricle lead is in place. Two J-shaped guidewires were parked in the inferior vena cava. B. The coronary sinus sheath is placed in the right atrium. Using electrophysiology catheter, the ostium of the coronary sinus is located. C. Cannulation of the coronary sinus using the electrophysiology catheter. D. The coronary sinus sheath is advanced over the electrophysiology catheter into the coronary sinus.

6.5 Target vessel

In the majority of cases, we successfully cannulate the CS. Our next step in LV lead placement is choosing the target vessel. How do we perform that? The vein is selected by performing the venogram of the CS (with or without CS balloon) in the left anterior oblique 30° projection.

The target area for LV lead placement is posterolateral or lateral branches.

There could be cases without any branch in posterolateral or lateral area. What to do in such a case? We aim for anterolateral branches. Rarely, but there could be cases where there are no suitable vessels for LV lead placement. The cause could be a complete absence of the branches or the presence of very small branches. What to do in such a case? We have at least two options: epicardial implantation of the bipolar lead on the LV lateral wall or consider LBB area pacing.

It is necessary to keep in mind that epicardial leads or LBB area pacing leads are bipolar only and, thereby, cannot be directly connected to quadripolar devices. This is why we always keep in our hospital a CRT device with a bipolar LV lead port.

How do you insert the lead into the target vein? We cannulate the target branch with 0.014-inch floppy wire and advance the LV lead over the wire.

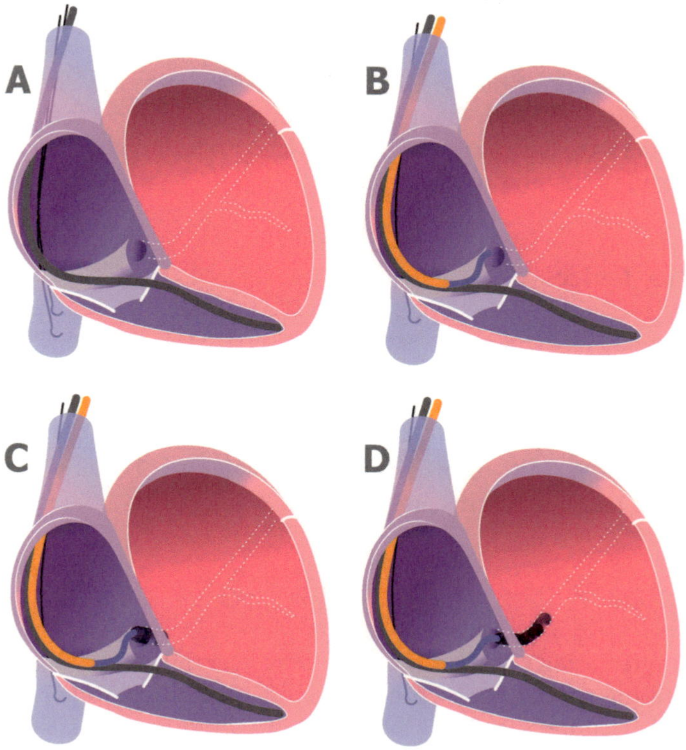

Figure 3.
Coronary sinus cannulation using telescopic method. A. The right ventricle lead is in place. B. The coronary sinus sheath is placed in the right atrium. The AL2 or AL3 catheter is advanced to reach the coronary sinus ostium. C. Some contrast is injected to confirm the engagement of the coronary sinus ostium. D. More contrast is used to confirm stable position. After that, the J shaped guidewire could be inserted deep into the coronary sinus.

Sometimes, the cannulation of the target branch is challenging due to the angulation of the vessel. In such a case, we can use an angiographic catheter (e.g., a 4F vertebral catheter) to cannulate that branch and send the floppy inside.

You must keep in mind that in some difficult cases there is not enough stability of the CS sheath to deliver the LV lead. In that case, we could solve the issue using extra support 0.014 ich floppy guidewires to send the LV lead in the target vein.

6.6 Types of the leads

What type of lead to choose?

There are several types, but experienced operators keep in mind some basic things.

If we are talking about CRT-D devices, a question about the number of coils in RV lead will arise. What is the best choice, single coil RV lead or dual coil RV lead?

For RV is advisable to use only single coil RV leads. The current evidence is that there are no additional benefits to the use of dual coil RV leads, and additional difficulties could arise if RV explantation is necessary in case of device infection [12, 13].

What about bipolar vs. quadripolar LV leads for CRT?

Quadripolar LV lead is the preferred choice with well-known advantages [14].

The use of the quadripolar LV leads offers much more vector possibilities for LV pacing. We could choose the vector with the lowest threshold, which will save battery life. We can change the vector if there is diaphragmatic stimulation or if there is loss of LV capture.

What about the shape of the LV lead? There are many types of LV lead shapes on the market: straight, S shape, L shape, etc. One of the best shapes for LV leads is the S shape. It permits us to have easy access of the lead to the target branch and to have good stability after implantation.

7. Types of the devices

The devices could be divided into pacemakers, referred as CRT-P and defibrillators, referred as CRT-D. The CRT-D devices could deliver high-energy interventions called shocks to treat severe arrhythmias such as ventricular fibrillation or ventricular tachycardia.

The devices could be MRI-compatible or not. They could be with bipolar LV leads or quadripolar LV leads, as was discussed earlier.

8. Complications

The CRT implantation could be a cause of many complications. Some of the complications could appear during procedure, and some are postoperative.

During the procedure, the physician must be attentive to avoid CS dissection or rupture, cardiac tamponade, and hemodynamic instability.

In the postoperative period, we have to avoid and to early detect and treat complications such as pocket hematoma, lead dislodgement, and pocket infection.

8.1 Hematoma

The pocket hematoma increases the risk for subsequent pocket infection [4]. The Bridge or Continue Coumadin for Device Surgery Randomized Controlled Trial (BRUISE CONTROL) proved that pocket hematoma is an independent risk factor for subsequent device infection [15].

Therefore, it is of utmost importance to avoid postoperative pocket hematoma.

To do so, it is advisable to not use bridge therapy with anticoagulants [3]. As an option, electrocautery could be used to perform meticulous hemostasis. And if necessary, use 500–1000 mg local tranexamic acid to obtain hemostasis [16].

8.2 Coronary sinus dissection or rupture

CS dissection or rupture is a known major complication during LV lead implantation (**Figure 4**).

How to prevent CS dissection? Manipulate the CS sheath and the guidewires gently. Please do not introduce the contrast agent in CS with high pressure if the sheath is perpendicular to CS wall. Check first with a small amount of contrast.

What should we do if we have dissection or rupture? Just take into consideration that usually, after 3–4 weeks, the dissection or rupture is healed, so the procedure could be continued in the postponed session.

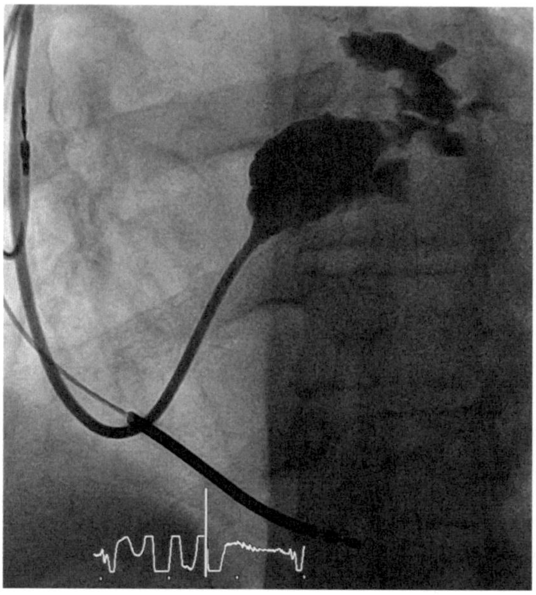

Figure 4.
Coronary sinus rupture. (Figure by Darciuc et al. [6], used under creative common attribution license).

8.3 Lead's dislodgement

To avoid lead dislodgement, it is preferable to use RA and RV leads with active fixation. Also, as we mentioned earlier, it is better to use S-shaped LV leads.

To avoid Twiddler syndrome, is important to secure the generator of the CRT-P or CRT-D inside the pocket.

We recommend that our patient avoid raising the elbow higher than the shoulder level at the surgery side for 6 weeks.

8.4 Free wall perforation and cardiac tamponade

Some patients could have apical aneurysms of the LV or very thin myocardium. Think about that when using the RV lead with active fixation. Consider securing the RV lead in septal region and avoid apical region.

8.5 Infection

Infection is an unpleasant complication, causing significant morbidity and mortality.

Infection rates are higher with device replacement or upgrade procedures [17]. As was reported by Olsen T. et al., the lifetime risk of system infection in patients with a pacemaker is 1.19%, with an implantable cardioverter defibrillator is 1.91%, with a CRT-P is 2.18%, and with a CRT-D is 3.35% [18].

To avoid infection, it is necessary to perform adequate patient preparation (antibiotic prophylaxis and skin preparation), use good surgical techniques, and avoid prolonged procedures to prevent hematoma formation (**Figure 5**).

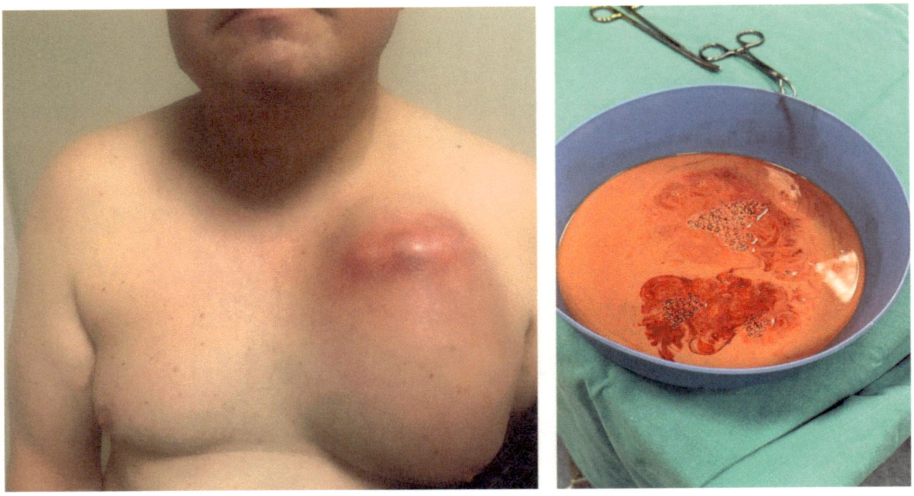

Figure 5.
Pocket infection. The cardiac resynchronization therapy device was implanted in 2019. The patient did not visit the device clinic for about 4 years. In 2023, he had a chest trauma, and a hematoma appeared in the region of the CRT-D generator. Thereafter, the hematoma became infected, and a phlegmon appeared. The system was successfully removed.

9. Follow-up

Is tremendously important to follow up with the patients.
During the follow-up visit, the physician:

- Is checking the appearance of the pocket.
- Is checking the percentage of biventricular pacing.
- Is performing CRT optimization by adjusting atrioventricular and ventriculo-ventricular delay. It could be performed using electrocardiography or echocardiography guidance.
- In CRT-D devices, is analyzing the events and the delivered therapies. Readjust the therapies as necessary.

10. Conclusions

CRT implantation is a challenging procedure that consists of many steps. Without proper planning and training, there could be challenges difficult to overcome.

EP specialists should have a backup plan for every single obstacle in CRT implantation.

It is important to develop the proper strategy to face all the challenges.

Acknowledgements

The author acknowledges the contribution to the current work of the previously published paper by Darciuc et al. [6], used under the Creative Common Attribution License.

DOI: http://dx.doi.org/10.5772/intechopen.1005119

Author details

Radu Darciuc
Cardiology Department, Medpark International Hospital, Chișinău,
Republic of Moldova

*Address all correspondence to: rdarciuc@yahoo.com

References

[1] Cazeau S, Ritter P, Bakdach S, Lazarus A, Limousin M, Henao L, et al. Four chamber pacing in dilated cardiomyopathy. Pacing and Clinical Electrophysiology. 1994;**17**(11 Pt. 2): 1974-1979. DOI: 10.1111/j.1540-8159.1994.tb03783.x

[2] Daubert JC, Ritter P, Le Breton H, Gras D, Leclercq C, Lazarus A, et al. Permanent left ventricular pacing with transvenous leads inserted into the coronary veins. Pacing and Clinical Electrophysiology. 1998;**21**(1 Pt. 2):239-245. DOI: 10.1111/j.1540-8159.1998.tb01096.x

[3] AlTurki A, Proietti R, Birnie DH, Essebag V. Management of antithrombotic therapy during cardiac implantable device surgery. Journal of Arrhythmia. 2016;**32**(3):163-169. DOI: 10.1016/j.joa.2015.12.003

[4] Glikson M, Nielsen JC, Kronborg MB, et al. 2021 ESC guidelines on cardiac pacing and cardiac resynchronization therapy [published correction appears in Eur Heart J. 2022 May 1;43(17):1651]. European Heart Journal. 2021;**42**(35):3427-3520. DOI: 10.1093/eurheartj/ehab364

[5] Birnie DH, Wang J, Alings M, et al. Risk factors for infections involving cardiac implanted electronic devices [published correction appears in J Am Coll Cardiol. 2020 Feb 25;75(7):840-841] [published correction appears in J Am Coll Cardiol. 2020 Aug 11;76(6):762]. Journal of the American College of Cardiology. 2019;**74**(23):2845-2854. DOI: 10.1016/j.jacc.2019.09.060

[6] Darciuc R, Boiciuc I, Ivanov D, Eraslan H, Batrinac A, Diker E. Technique of the cardiac resynchronization therapy device implantation. Medical Research Archives. 2023;**11**(7.1). DOI: 10.18103/mra.v11i7.1.4057

[7] Burri H, Sunthorn H, Dorsaz PA, Shah D. Prospective study of axillary vein puncture with or without contrast venography for pacemaker and defibrillator lead implantation. Pacing and Clinical Electrophysiology. 2005;**28**(Suppl. 1):S280-S283. DOI: 10.1111/j.1540-8159.2005.00039.x

[8] Cheng CM, Huang JL, Wu TJ, et al. Novel tips for engaging the coronary sinus guided by right ventricular lead. Europace. 2012;**14**(12):1754-1758. DOI: 10.1093/europace/eus192

[9] Gunes H, Aksu E, Nacar H, Kerkutluoglu M, Gunes H, Ozgul S. What is the most appropriate method for coronary sinus cannulation? The telescopic method or the electrophysiologic method? PLoS One. 2018;**13**(9):e0203534. Published 2018 Sep 14. DOI: 10.1371/journal.pone.0203534

[10] Katritsis DG. A novel technique for placement of coronary sinus pacing leads in cardiac resynchronization therapy. Europace. 2007;**9**(10):878-879. DOI: 10.1093/europace/eum146

[11] Worley SJ. Challenging implants require tools and techniques not tips and tricks. Cardiac Electrophysiology Clinics. 2019;**11**(1):75-87. DOI: 10.1016/j.ccep.2018.11.003

[12] Aoukar PS, Poole JE, Johnson GW, et al. No benefit of a dual coil over a single coil ICD lead: Evidence from the sudden cardiac death in heart failure trial. Heart Rhythm. 2013;**10**(7):970-976. DOI: 10.1016/j.hrthm.2013.03.046

[13] Sunderland N, Kaura A, Murgatroyd F, Dhillon P, Scott PA. Outcomes with single-coil versus dual-coil implantable cardioverter defibrillators: A meta-analysis. Europace. 2018;**20**(3):e21-e29. DOI: 10.1093/europace/euw438

[14] Rijal S, Wolfe J, Rattan R, et al. Lead related complications in quadripolar versus bipolar left ventricular leads. Indian Pacing and Electrophysiology Journal. 2017;**17**(1):3-7. DOI: 10.1016/j.ipej.2016.10.008

[15] Essebag V, Verma A, Healey JS, Krahn AD, Kalfon E, Coutu B, et al. Clinically significant pocket hematoma increases long-term risk of device infection: Bruise control infection study. Journal of the American College of Cardiology. 2016;**67**(11):1300-1308. DOI: 10.1016/j.jacc.2016.01.009

[16] Beton O, Saricam E, Kaya H, et al. Bleeding complications during cardiac electronic device implantation in patients receiving antithrombotic therapy: Is there any value of local tranexamic acid? BMC Cardiovascular Disorders. 2016;**16**:73. Published 2016 Apr 22. DOI: 10.1186/s12872-016-0251-1

[17] Rattanawong P, Kewcharoen J, Mekraksakit P, Mekritthikrai R, Prasitlumkum N, Vutthikraivit W, et al. Device infections in implantable cardioverter defibrillators versus permanent pacemakers: A systematic review and meta-analysis. Journal of Cardiovascular Electrophysiology. 2019;**30**(7):1053-1065. DOI: 10.1111/jce.13932

[18] Olsen T, Jørgensen OD, Nielsen JC, Thøgersen AM, Philbert BT, Johansen JB. Incidence of device-related infection in 97 750 patients: Clinical data from the complete Danish device-cohort (1982-2018). European Heart Journal. 2019;**40**(23):1862-1869. DOI: 10.1093/eurheartj/ehz316

Chapter 6

Cardiac Resynchronization Therapy: With or without Defibrillation

Somshukla Ghosh, Rabya S. Saraf and Ahmed Hussein

Abstract

Approximately one-third of patients with cardiomyopathy and heart failure (HF) have intraventricular dyssynchrony that leads to progression of left ventricular (LV) systolic dysfunction and HF symptoms. In these patients, the use of cardiac resynchronization therapy (CRT) can result in improved LV function and favorable cardiac remodeling. These structural changes were found to result in a reduction in mortality. As such, it could be postulated that CRT device, without a defibrillator (CRT-P), may be enough to reduce mortality in these patients. Conversely, defibrillators without CRT have been used for the purpose of mortality reduction in the same group of patients. In an attempt to answer the question about the best device to be used for mortality reduction in these patients, we studied the clinical trials that compared the reduction in mortality benefit in patients with cardiomyopathy and HF with the use of CRT-P, ICD alone, and CRT in combination with ICD (CRT-D).

Keywords: cardiac resynchronization therapy, systolic heart failure, defibrillation therapy, COMPANION, RAFT, MADIT-CRT

1. Introduction

Cardiac resynchronization therapy (CRT) is a type of cardiac pacing that was introduced in 1990s with the aim to achieve simultaneous or near simultaneous activation of the left and right ventricles to reduce ventricular dyssynchrony, which has been known to cause progression of LV systolic dysfunction and clinical heart failure (HF) [1]. In normal myocardium, the electrical waveform that travels through the conduction system is uniform and ensures synchronized depolarization of the ventricles. In diseased myocardium, areas of delayed conduction and activation are seen due to damage to the conduction fibers as well as changes to the electrochemical substrate [2]. This delay in conduction will manifest as QRS prolongation on an electrocardiogram and therefore is a clue to the presence of electrical dyssynchrony.

Electrical dyssynchrony can result in mechanical dyssynchrony, which can exhibit in three different ways: interventricular dyssynchrony, intraventricular dyssynchrony, and atrioventricular dyssynchrony. One of the consequences of long-standing dyssynchrony is cardiac remodeling, which often worsens clinical outcomes [3].

There have been multiple observational studies that have demonstrated an association between electrical dyssynchrony and adverse clinical outcomes. Approximately one-third of patients with advanced heart failure have prolonged QRS duration, indicating electrical ventricular dyssynchrony, and these patients have an increased risk of adverse outcomes [4].

In patients with heart failure due to cardiomyopathy and evidence of electromechanical ventricular dyssynchrony, CRT exerts beneficial effects by improving dyssynchrony, thus restoring the physiologic atrioventricular relationship, which in turn results in improved myocardial oxygen consumption, LV function, favorable cardiac remodeling, and reduced severity of mitral regurgitation [3, 4]. These structural changes of CRT translated into clinical benefits noted in appropriately selected patients including functional improvement in exercise capacity, improved quality of life, and a reduction in heart failure admissions and mortality. Therefore, it has been postulated that stand-alone CRT (CRT-P) may be enough to reduce mortality without the need for an added defibrillation therapy. On the other hand, defibrillation therapy using ICDs alone had been used for almost a decade before the introduction of CRT and was proven to reduce mortality in patients with heart failure due to cardiomyopathy, both with and without evidence electromechanical ventricular dyssynchrony.

As noted in the current guidelines, there is significant overlap in the indications for CRT and ICD devices implantations in patients with cardiomyopathy and heart failure [5].

In the guidelines, the CRT indications include patients with left ventricular ejection fraction (LVEF) of 35% or less, who have been treated with goal-directed medical therapy for at least 90 days or 40 days, if cardiomyopathy occurred following myocardial infarction (MI), as potential candidates for CRT.

For patients who are NYHA class I, it is a class IIb recommendation for CRT if LVEF is 30% or less, and the electrocardiogram shows a QRS duration more than 150 msec and LBBB pattern, and the patient has ischemic cardiomyopathy. While in patients with LVEF of 35% or less, with NYHA class II-III symptoms, it is class I indication for CRT if QRS duration is 150 msec or more and there is an LBBB pattern and a class IIa indication for CRT if QRS duration is between 120 and 149 msec and there is an LBBB pattern.

According to the same guidelines, the primary prevention ICD indications bear similarities to the CRT indications as follows. ICD therapy is indicated as a Class I recommendation in patients with LVEF less than or equal to 35% due to prior MI who are at least 40 days post-MI and are in NYHA functional Class I-III. Also, ICD therapy is indicated as a Class I recommendation in patients with nonischemic cardiomyopathy who have an LVEF less than or equal to 35% and who are in NYHA functional Class II or III.

Whether an implantable cardioverter-defibrillator (ICD) should be combined with CRT is dependent on if the patient meets criteria for primary prevention as mentioned above, or secondary prevention in patients who have a history of ventricular arrhythmias without any identifiable reversible causes.

2. Studies that compared device therapy clinical outcomes

Several clinical trials compared the reduction in mortality benefit in patients with heart failure with the use of CRT-P, ICD alone, and CRT-D. In this chapter, we are summarizing the results of some of these trials.

2.1 The multicenter insync randomized clinical evaluation (MIRACLE) and the multicenter insync ICD randomized clinical evaluation (MIRACLE ICD) trial

Published in 2002, the double-blind, randomized MIRACLE trial sought to evaluate the effect of CRT as compared with no CRT on functional capacity and quality of life in patients with existing heart failure and known ventricular dyssynchrony. A secondary goal was to assess the safety of CRT in patients with HF. They hypothesized that CRT would resynchronize contraction of the failing LV and improve cardiac performance [6].

The study enrolled 453 patients; only 32 were female, with an average age of 64 years and NYHA Class III and IV symptoms who were followed for at least 6 months. The patient population had the following characteristics: LVEF <35%, QRS >130 msec, LV end-diastolic dimension >55 mm, and a six-minute walking distance of at least 450 meters. The primary endpoints were defined by a measure of quality of life (determined by the Minnesota Living With Heart Failure Questionnaire), NYHA functional class, and the six-minute hall walk.

After inclusion criteria were met and a baseline assessment completed, the participants underwent device and were randomized to either the control group (no CRT, n = 225) or CRT group (n = 228). They subsequently underwent follow-up at one, three, and six-months. The electrophysiologist was the only unblinded third party, and the rest of the team, which consisted of the heart failure specialist, the managing physician, and the patient, were blinded to study assignment during the six-month period. After the six-month follow-up period, patients in the control arm could go into the resynchronization mode.

Before randomization, all participants were required to be maintained on an angiotensin-converting enzyme inhibitor or ACE inhibitor substitute for 1 month and those on beta-blocker therapy were required to be on a stable regimen for at least 3 months before randomization. Changes to medical therapy were discouraged during the study.

The trial showed that in comparison with placebo, CRT was associated with significant improvement in the quality of life ($p = 0.001$), time on treadmill during exercise testing ($p = 0.001$), the six-minute walk distance ($p = 0.005$), NYHA class ($p < 0.001$), and EF ($p < 0.001$). Furthermore, the QRS duration was significantly lower in CRT patients compared with control ($p < 0.001$), as was the need for hospital admission ($p = 0.02$) and intravenous medication ($p = 0.004$). Using the Heart Failure Clinical Composite Outcome Measure, a larger percentage of CRT patients were classified as improved compared to the control group (67 vs. 39%, $p < 0.001$) and fewer were classified as worsened compared to the control group (16 vs. 27%). Death or worsening heart failure requiring hospitalization occurred less frequently in the CRT arm as well (28 vs. 44%, hazard ratio 0.60, 95% confidence interval 0.37–0.96; $p = 0.03$).

In conclusion, the MIRACLE trial demonstrated that biventricular pacing was associated with improved quality of life and functional class among patients with HF and ventricular dyssynchrony.

Subsequently, the MIRACLE-ICD trial was published in 2003 and aimed to compare the effect of CRT plus ICD versus ICD alone on the quality of life, functional capacity, and safety in patients with chronic heart failure and ventricular dyssynchrony [7].

The MIRACLE-ICD trial enrolled 369 patients, only 23 participants were female, with a mean age of 67 years with most of them categorized as NYHA class III and a small percentage as NYHA class IV, LVEF ≤35%, a QRS duration ≥130 msec, LV end-diastolic diameter ≥ 55 mm, and a stable drug regimen for at least 1 month. The participants included also had to have a history of cardiac arrest due to ventricular fibrillation or ventricular tachyarrhythmia, or spontaneously sustained ventricular tachyarrhythmia, or inducible ventricular fibrillation or sustained ventricular tachyarrhythmia.

The primary end points included NYHA functional class, quality of life score, and distance covered during the six-minute walking test. All patients underwent device implantation after baseline assessment and were randomized to either the control group (CRT off, ICD on, n = 182) or experimental group (CRT and ICD both on, n = 187) and followed for 6 months. The electrophysiologist served as the unblinded third party, and the rest of the managing team was blinded. Compared with placebo, CRT was associated with a significant improvement in NYHA class by at least one class (median class change −1 vs. 0, p = 0.007) and quality of life (−17.5 vs. −11 points, p = 0.02), but there was no difference in the 6-minute walk distance.

In addition, multiple secondary end points were improved in the CRT arm, although not all with significant p-values, including time on the treadmill during exercise testing, improved end-diastolic and end-systolic volumes, and ejection fraction. There was also a trend for a higher percentage of CRT patients to be classified as improved using the change in overall clinical status. There was no difference in mortality or the composite of death or repeat hospitalization for worsening HF.

2.2 The comparison of medical therapy, pacing, and defibrillation in heart failure (COMPANION) trial

The COMPANION trial was published in 2004 and was the first randomized, controlled trial that compared optimized pharmacological therapy, CRT delivered with a biventricular pacemaker (CRT-P), and CRT with defibrillator (CRT-D) in patients with advanced chronic heart failure. The trial was conducted at 128 U.S. centers between early 2000 and end of 2002 and included 1520 patients with New York Heart Association (NYHA) class III or IV heart failure (which could be ischemic or nonischemic in etiology), LVEF <35%, and a QRS duration of more than 120 msec [8].

These patients were randomized in a 1:2:2 ratio to receive optimized medical therapy (diuretics, angiotensin-converting-enzyme inhibitor, beta-blocker, and mineralocorticoid receptor antagonist) alone or in combination with CRT or CRT-D. The primary composite end point was the time to death from any cause or hospitalization for any cause. Secondary outcome was death from any cause. The median follow-up duration was about 14 months. Of the enrolled patients, mean age was 67 years, about one-third were female, 85% had NYHA class III heart failure, and mean EF was 22%.

Compared to the arm where patients where receiving optimized medical therapy only, patients with CRT and CRT-D had improved primary end point by 34% and 40%, respectively. CRT reduced the risk of the secondary end point of death from any cause by 24%, and CRT-D reduced the risk by 36%. All data was statistically significant. There was an even larger reduction in the outcome of death from or hospitalization for heart failure. It is noteworthy that in both CRT and CRT-D arms, lowering of the hazard ratio was directly proportional to an increasing QRS interval.

2.3 The multicenter automatic defibrillator implantation (the MADIT-CRT) trial

The MADIT-CRT was published in 2009 and was designed to determine whether CRT would improve clinical outcomes (specifically death and heart failure events) in patients with LVEF <30% (ischemic or nonischemic cardiomyopathy), QRS duration of at least 130 ms, but with milder cardiac symptoms (NYHA I and II) [7]. Patients were randomized in a 3:2 ratio to receive CRT-D (1089 patients) or ICD alone (731 patients). All patients were on goal-directed medical therapy (diuretics, angiotensin-converting-enzyme inhibitor, beta-blocker, mineralocorticoid antagonist). The primary end point was death from any cause or a nonfatal heart-failure event. During an average follow up of 2.4 years, the patients in the CRT-D group had a lower rate of the primary outcome with 35% relative reduction in all-cause mortality ($p = 0.048$) and a 63% relative reduction in first heart failure event ($p < 0.001$).

Echocardiography was performed at baseline and at the 1-year follow-up to assess changes in LV volumes and ejection fraction in the two study groups. There was reduction in LV volumes and significant increment in the ejection fraction in patients in the CRT-D group as compared to the those in the ICD group.

When subgroup analysis of the primary outcome was performed, it revealed that women benefitted more than men from CRT-D and that the benefit of CRT-D over ICD was seen only in patients who had QRS duration of more than 150 msec.

The median age of patients enrolled in the COMPANION and MADIT-CRT trials was 67 and 65 years, respectively. Therefore, the benefit of CRT in older patients with heart failure with reduced ejection fraction (HFrEF) was not adequately assessed.

A recently published retrospective study has looked at whether CRT benefited patients with HFrEF who were older than 65 years [9]. Patients were categorized by age (65–74, 75–84, and 85+ years), and they had undergone implantation of CRT-D or ICD device between 2008 and 2015. The risk of death was lower in the CRT-D group by 10% and 18% in the age groups of 75–84 and 85 + years, respectively. This supports the use of CRT in older patients undergoing ICD implantation.

2.4 Resynchronization reverses remodeling in systolic left ventricular dysfunction (REVERSE trial)

In the large multicenter, randomized, double-blind REVERSE trial, which was published in 2008, participants were randomized to have their CRT-D turned on for 1 year and then CRT-D turned off for 1 year or vice versa [10].

They studied a total of 610 patients with NYHA functional class I or II heart failure, a QRS >120 msec, and an LVEF <40% who were randomly assigned to active CRT (CRT-ON; $n = 419$) or control (CRT-OFF; $n = 191$) for 12 months. The primary end point was the HF clinical composite response and was scored as improved, unchanged, or worsened based on how the patients did over 12 months. In the CRT-ON group, there was only 16% worsening in the HF clinical composite response as compared with 21% in the CRT-OFF group ($p = 0.10$).

In addition, patients assigned to CRT-ON experienced a greater improvement in LV end-systolic volume index ($p < 0.0001$) and other measures of LV remodeling, and they had a significantly delayed time-to-first HF hospitalization (hazard ratio: 0.47, $p = 0.03$).

The concept of reverse remodeling by CRT has been described in small studies with a 6-month follow-up prior to the REVERSE trial, but it was reinforced with the much larger REVERSE trial with a longer follow-up period [11, 12].

Overall, the REVERSE trial demonstrated that CRT, in combination with optimal medical therapy (with or without defibrillator), reduced the risk for heart failure hospitalizations and improved ventricular structure and function in patients with mild HF symptoms or those who were asymptomatic, that is, NYHA functional class II and I, respectively.

2.5 Resynchronization-defibrillation for ambulatory heart failure (RAFT) trial

Published in 2010, the multicenter RAFT trial studied 1798 patients with NYHA class II or III heart failure, intrinsic QRS duration ≥120 msec or a paced QRS duration ≥200 msec, and LVEF ≤30% (ischemic or nonischemic etiology). These patients were randomized to receive either CRT-D or ICD alone. The primary outcome was mortality and hospitalization for HF with a mean follow-up duration of 40 months. The primary outcome occurred in 25% lesser patients in the CRT-D group than in the ICD group. The number needed to treat was exceptionally low at only 14. However, patients in the CRT-D group had a significantly higher adverse event rate as compared to the ICD group [13].

The probability of event-free survival at 5 years was 8.9% more in the CRT-D group than in the ICD group, while the probability of survival at 5 years was 6% more in the CRT-D group than in the ICD group.

Only 20% of patients in this trial had NYHA class III heart failure; however, on subgroup analysis, similar reductions in the risk of death or hospitalization for heart failure were observed in the two study arms. Approximately 70% of the patients had LBBB type of QRS morphology, and these patients benefitted at a greater degree than those with nonspecific interventricular conduction delay. Furthermore, CRT-D was found to be more beneficial for patients with intrinsic QRS duration >150 msec.

The RAFT Long-Term Study followed the patients in the RAFT trial for a mean 7.7 years to study the effect of CRT on long-term survival [14]. 1050 patients of the total 1798 patients were included in this trial. Among these patients with reduced EF, widened QRS complex, and NYHA class II or III HF, the survival benefit associated with CRT-D as compared with ICD was sustained during a median of nearly 14 years of follow-up [14].

2.6 Cardiac resynchrnization therapy upgrade in heart failure with right ventricular pacing (budapest CRT upgrade trial)

The Budapest CRT Upgrade trial, presented at ESC Congress 2023, showed that upgradation to CRT-D from pacemaker or ICD in patients with ejection fraction (EF) less than 35%, QRS duration ≥150 msec, and RV pacing burden of ≥20% resulted in decreased all-cause mortality, hospitalization from heart failure, and decreased end-systolic volume.

A total of 360 patients with EF ≤ 35% (NYHA heart failure symptoms II-Iva) on goal-directed medical therapy who had undergone implantation of a pacemaker or ICD ≥ 6 months prior and had a wide QRS duration ≥150 msec with pacing burden of ≥20% were randomized in 3:2 ratio to a CRT-D upgrade group and an ICD group. During a median follow-up of more than a year, the primary outcome of a composite of hospitalization from heart failure, all-cause mortality and decreased reverse LV modeling occurred in 32.4% patients in the CRT-D arm and 78.9% patients in the ICD arm, $p < 0.0001$. The number needed to treat was incredibly low at 2.2. Notably, the occurrence of ventricular arrhythmia was substantially lower in the CRT-D group. Procedure or device-related complications were comparable in the 2 groups.

3. For patients with cardiomyopathy and heart failure, which device to implant: ICD, CRT, or CRT-D?

Meta-analysis of the studies discussed above provided strong evidence that CRT reduces mortality and hospitalization and improves cardiac function and structure in symptomatic HF patients on OPT with severely depressed LVEF (i.e., ≤35%) and complete LBBB. In these patients, CRT was superior either to optimal medical therapy or to ICD alone. Also, analysis of these studies demonstrated that CRT-D provided a slightly better degree of reduction in mortality with a trade-off of higher cost and to some degree higher procedural complications (**Table 1**) [15].

In patients indicated for CRT, defibrillation therapy is typically deferred in patients with life expectancy less than a year, NYHA Class IV, severe renal disease and other severe comorbidities, cachexia, and frailty (**Table 2**) [15].

	CRT-D	CRT-P
Mortality reduction	Similar level of evidence but CRT-D slightly better	Similar level of evidence but CRT-P slightly worse
Complications	Higher	Lower
Costs	Higher	Lower

CRT-D = cardiac resynchronization therapy and defibrillator; and CRT-P = cardiac resynchronization therapy and pacemaker.

Table 1.
Comparative results of CRT-D vs. CRT-P in primary preventions.

Factors favoring CRT-P	Factors favoring CRT-D
Advanced heart failure	Life expectancy >1 year
Severe renal insufficiency or dialysis	Stable heart failure, NYHA II
Other major co-morbidities	Ischaemic heart disease (low and intermediate MADIT risk score)
Frailty	Lack of comorbidities
Cachexia	

CRT-D = cardiac resynchronization therapy and defibrillator; CRT-P = cardiac resynchronization therapy and pacemaker; MADIT = Multicentre Automatic Defibrillator Trial; and NYHA = New York Heart Association.

Table 2.
Clinical guidance to the choice of CRT-P or CRT-D in primary prevention.

4. Pacing site-dependent arrhythmia

This phenomenon was described by Medina-Ravell et al. in 2003 and was defined as an arrhythmia due to simultaneous pacing of right ventricle (RV) endocardium and LV epicardium [16]. Normally, ventricle activation starts at the endocardium and spreads through the myocardium to the epicardium. Therefore, LV epicardial pacing alters ventricular activation and repolarization dynamics, which leads to QT interval prolongation rendering the ventricle vulnerable to extrasystoles that result in R on T phenomenon, Torsades des Pointes, or non-sustained or sustained polymorphic ventricular tachycardia. The incidence of this condition was reported to be about 4% and mostly occurred in ischemic cardiomyopathy patients [17].

Because about 4% of CRT implant patients could die soon after device implantation due to the device-related arrhythmia described above if left untreated, CRT-D is preferably selected instead CRT-P when a patient meets CRT indications.

5. Future prospective

None of the randomized controlled trials for either CRT or CRT-D had the patients on goal-directed medical therapy optimized as per present day guidelines. These trials had majority of patients on beta-blockers, but the proportion of patients on mineralocorticoid receptor antagonist or angiotensin convertase inhibitors/angiotensin receptor blockers was much less. The role of angiotensin receptor/neprilysin inhibitor and SGLT-2 inhibitors in heart failure treatment were yet not established when these trials were conducted. Hence, there is a scope for newer trials to be conducted with patients on optimized goal-directed medical therapy as per present day guidelines.

Also, left ventricular scarring may lead to ineffective CRT. Cardiac MRI is the current gold standard for detecting myocardial scarring. With the use of cardiac MRI, it may be helpful in guiding LV lead deployment. The strategy of avoiding myocardial scar during LV lead implantation has not been studied in a multicenter, randomized, controlled trials because of the difficulty in including a control group not treated with CRT. Cardiac MRI can also provide measurements of global and segmental cardiac function and permit localization and quantification of myocardial perfusion. These measures provide important information on the cause and prognosis of patients with heart failure. Therefore, further studies regarding the use of cardiac MRI to select appropriate candidates for CRT and to achieve the maximum benefit from it are needed [18].

Another potential benefit of cardiac MRI use in selection of the device relates to myocardial scar as a possible predictor of arrhythmic events. Some studies showed that scar burden is a more powerful predictor of SCD than LVEF. For example, in the MADIT-II (Multicenter Automatic Defibrillator Implantation Trial II) trial, the extent of fixed perfusion defects on nuclear imaging was a strong predictor of lethal arrhythmias over a follow-up of 30 months [19]. As such, the presence of extensive myocardial scarring in patients eligible for CRT may be a good reason to favor the use of CRT-D over CRT-P in these patients.

6. Conclusion

In the presence of QRS duration of ≥150 msec and LBBB in patients with cardiomyopathy and reduced ejection fraction LVEF of ≤35%, and in the absence of contraindications for defibrillation therapy, it is suggested that the maximum reduction of mortality benefit may be achieved with the use of CRT-D device, possibly due to decreased risk of death due to arrhythmia with this combination.

Nevertheless, CRT-P has proven benefits that do not only include improvement in heart failure symptoms and quality of life, but include significant mortality reduction benefit as well and therefore can still be used when defibrillation therapy is contraindicated.

Author details

Somshukla Ghosh, Rabya S. Saraf and Ahmed Hussein*
Saint Louis University School of Medicine, SSM Health/Saint Louis University Hospital, Saint Louis, Missouri, USA

*Address all correspondence to: ahmed_abdellatif_hussein@yahoo.co.uk

References

[1] Dan GA. 2021 ESC guidelines on cardiac pacing and cardiac resynchronisation therapy. European Society of Cardiology. 2021;**16**:e55. DOI: 10.15420/ecr.2021.51

[2] Shenkman HJ, Pampati V, Khandelwal AK, et al. Congestive heart failure and QRS duration: Establishing prognosis study. Chest. 2002;**122**(2):528-534

[3] Jaffe LM, Morin DP. Cardiac resynchronization therapy: History, present status, and future directions. The Ochsner Journal. 2014;**14**(4):596-607

[4] Iuliano S, Fisher SG, Karasik PE, Fletcher RD, Singh SN. Department of Veterans Affairs Survival Trial of antiarrhythmic therapy in congestive heart failure. QRS duration and mortality in patients with congestive heart failure. American Heart Journal. 2002;**143**(6):1085-1091. DOI: 10.1067/mhj.2002.122516

[5] Tracy CM, Epstein AE, Darbar D, Dimarco JP, Dunbar SB, Estes NAM, et al. 2012 ACCF/AHA/HRS focused update incorporated into the ACCF/AHA/HRS 2008 guidelines for device-based therapy of cardiac rhythm abnormalities: A report of the American college of cardiology foundation/American heart association task force on practice guidelines and the heart rhythm society. Journal of the American College of Cardiology. 2013;**61**(3):e6-e75. DOI: 10.1016/j.jacc.2012.11.007

[6] Abraham WT, Young JB, Leon AR, et al. Effects of cardiac resynchronization on disease progression in patients with left ventricular systolic dysfunction, an indication for an implantable cardioverter defibrillator, and mildly symptomatic chronic heart failure. Circulation. 2004;**110**:2864-2868

[7] Moss AJ, Hall WJ, Cannom DS, Klein H, Brown MW, Daubert JP, et al. Cardiac-resynchronization therapy for the prevention of heart-failure events. The New England Journal of Medicine. 2009;**361**(14):1329-1338. DOI: 10.1056/NEJMoa0906431. Epub. 2009 Sep 1

[8] Bristow MR, Saxon LA, Boehmer J, Krueger S, Kass DA, De Marco T, et al. Cardiac-resynchronization therapy with or without an implantable defibrillator in advanced chronic heart failure. The New England Journal of Medicine. 2004;**350**(21):2140-2150. DOI: 10.1056/NEJMoa032423

[9] Zeitler EP, Austin AM, Leggett CG, Gilstrap LG, Friedman DJ, Skinner JS, et al. Complications and mortality following CRT-D versus ICD implants in older medicare beneficiaries with heart failure. JACC Heart Failure. 2022;**10**(3):147-157. DOI: 10.1016/j.jchf.2021.10.012. Epub. 2022 Jan 12

[10] Linde C, Abraham WT, Gold MR, St. John Sutton M, Ghio S, Daubert C, et al. Randomized trial of cardiac resynchronization in mildly symptomatic heart failure patients and in asymptomatic patients with left ventricular dysfunction and previous heart failure symptoms. Journal of the American College of Cardiology. 2008;**52**(23):1834-1843. DOI: 10.1016/j.jacc.2008.08.027. Epub. 2008 Nov 7

[11] Abraham WT, Fisher WG, Smith AL, Delurgio DB, Leon AR, Loh E, et al. Cardiac resynchronization in chronic heart failure. The New England Journal of Medicine. 2002;**346**(24):1845-1853. DOI: 10.1056/NEJMoa013168

[12] Higgins SL, Hummel JD, Niazi IK, et al. Cardiac resynchronization therapy for the treatment of heart failure in patients with intraventricular conduction delay and malignant ventricular tachyarrhythmias. Journal of the American College of Cardiology. 2003;**42**(8):1454-1459

[13] Tang AS, Wells GA, Talajic M, Arnold MO, Sheldon R, Connolly S, et al. Cardiac-resynchronization therapy for mild-to-moderate heart failure. The New England Journal of Medicine. 2010;**363**(25):2385-2395. DOI: 10.1056/NEJMoa1009540. Epub. 2010 Nov 14

[14] Sapp JL, Sivakumaran S, Redpath CJ, Khan H, Parkash R, Exner DV, et al. Long-term outcomes of resynchronization-defibrillation for heart failure. The New England Journal of Medicine. 2024;**390**(3):212-220. DOI: 10.1056/NEJMoa2304542

[15] Brignole M, Auricchio A, Baron-Esquivias G, Bordachar P, Boriani G, Breithardt O-A, et al. ESC guidelines on cardiac pacing and cardiac resynchronization therapy: The task force on cardiac pacing and resynchronization therapy of the European Society of Cardiology (ESC). Developed in collaboration with the European Heart Rhythm Association. European Heart Journal. 2013, 2013;**15**(8):1070-1118. DOI: 10.1093/EUROPACE/EUT206

[16] Medina-Ravell VA, Lankipalli RS, Yan GX, Antzelevitch C, Medina-Malpica NA, Medina-Malpica OA, et al. Effect of epicardial or biventricular pacing to prolong QT interval and increase transmural dispersion of repolarization: Does resynchronization therapy pose a risk for patients predisposed to long QT or torsade de pointes? Circulation. 2003;**107**:740-746

[17] Shukla G, Chaudhry GM, Orlov M, Hoffmeister P, Haffajee C. Potential proarrhythmic effect of biventricular pacing: Fact or myth? Heart Rhythm. 2005;**2**:951-956

[18] Leyva F. The role of cardiovascular magnetic resonance in cardiac resynchronization therapy. Heart Failure Clinics. 2017;**13**(1):63-77

[19] Morishima T, Sone HT, et al. Risk stratification of patients with prior myocardial infarction and advanced left ventricular dysfunction by gated myocardial perfusion SPECT imaging. Journal of Nuclear Cardiology. 2008;**15**:631-637